THE
CUPS AND SCALES
EVERYTHING
WEIGHED &
MEASURED
COOKBOOK

7 Sample Plans of Eating and 300 Recipes - No Sugar, Wheat, Flour - With and Without Starches and Grains

People and Groups

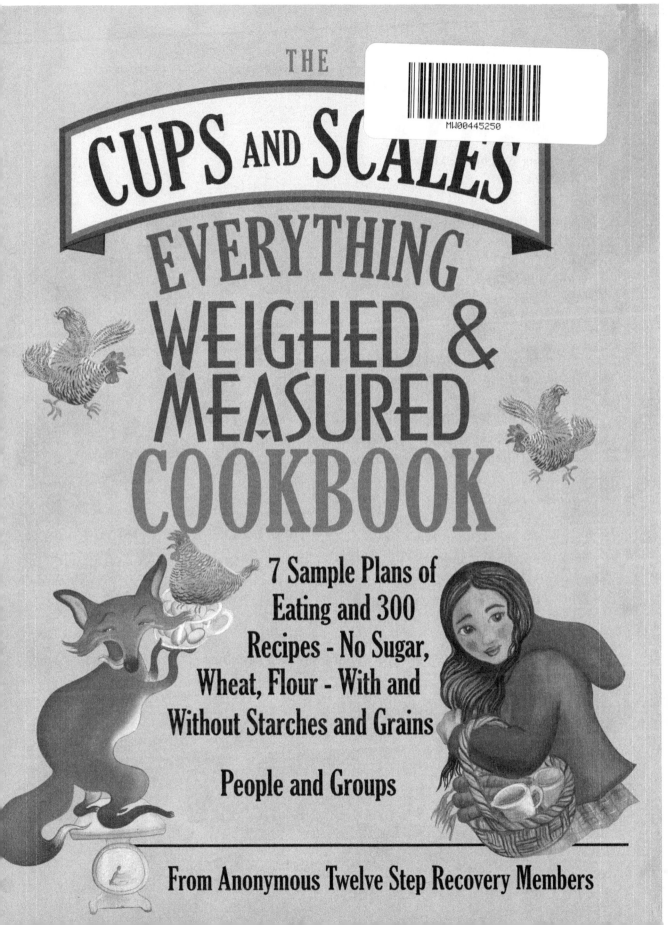

From Anonymous Twelve Step Recovery Members

The
Cups & Scales
Everything Weighed & Measured
Cookbook

7 Sample Plans of Eating &
300 Recipes - No Sugar,
Wheat, Flour - With and
Without Starches and Grains

People and Groups

By Anonymous Twelve Step Recovery Members
Illustrations by Mercedes McDonald

Cover Design: Cheryl Klinginsmith
© 2011 Text: Partnerships for Community
© 2011 Illustrations: Mercedes McDonald

Partnerships for Community
561 Hudson Street, Suite 23
New York, N.Y. 10014
Printed in United States

Library of Congress Cataloguing in Publication Data Pending
ISBN: 1-933639-94-6
ISBN: 978-1-933639-94-9

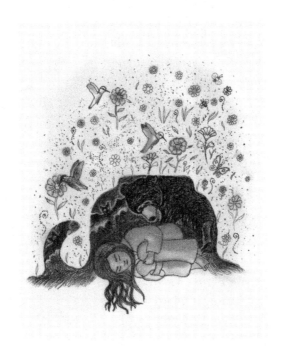

I may not want to use the tools
available to me.
Not yet.

I HAVE A SPIRIT FRIEND.
HOPE EXISTS.

TABLE OF CONTENTS

Introduction

The Cups & Scales Everything Weighed & Measured Cookbook is a factual and inspirational guide. It contains *7 Sample Plans of Eating and 300 Recipes - No Sugar, Wheat, Flour - With and Without Starches and Grains - Everything Weighed & Measured.*

- Find *Sample Plans of Eating*. View seven sample plans of eating - plans with one fruit to four fruits per day, and plans with and without starches and grains. Use the recipes in this book separately or in combination with a plan of eating. See websites where you can obtain plans of eating supported by non-profit overeating and food addiction groups. Read an essay on *Facing Plan of Eating Choices with My Healthcare Practitioner & A Sponsor* from a Twelve Step Recovery member.

- Learn about adjustable *Frequencies of Meals*.

- See over *300 Recipes - No Sugar-Wheat-Flour - Everything Weighed and Measured, With and Without Starches and Grains*. Recipes may be used in combination with the plans of eating.

- See *What's In It - What Isn't In It,* ingredients used in the recipes, and "what" a serving amount is in the ingredients and foods.

- Read *To Weigh & Measure or To Not Weigh & Measure* and learn about *The Phenomenon of Weighing & Measuring*.

- Hear one contributor's take on *The Benefits. I Eat with Safety & Security* Because I Shop for the Right Foods & Weigh and Measure
  - 'I Cook & Eat With Happiness'
  - 'I Cook & Eat Without Remorse'
  - 'I Get Consistent Brain Functioning & Balanced Metabolism'
  - 'I Get 'Peace of Mind on a Plate"
  - 'I am safe'
  - 'I have never lost the right to eat'
  - 'I have another meal coming'
  - 'I have the comfort of knowing where I will get my next meal'
  - 'I have the safety, security & comfort of knowing what will be in it'
  - 'I use cups and scales for my better ordering and preservation'
  - 'I get clarity and understanding'

- Get information on *People & Groups* who offer support in letting go of compulsive eating, including people in *Compulsive Overeaters Anonymous-HOW. Cups & Scales Forum; Food Addicts Anonymous; Food Addicts: The Body Knows Online Discussion Group; Greysheeter's Anonymous; Overeaters Anonymous, regular OA meetings and OA H.O.W .and 90-Day meetings; and Recovery from Food Addiction*. Contacts are willing to be your phone buddy or to sponsor you. Get access in this book to free phone meeting numbers, websites, and email addresses to contact people and groups.

- Read an essay on *The 'Science & Spirit' of Meals vs. Pounce & Grazing,* by a Twelve Step Recovery Member.
- Think about *Sweeteners: Each One Makes a Decision* , an essay by a Twelve Step Recovery member, including a brief history of sugar.
- See *Resources and Links* to products some of us use, including cups & scales, non-aerosol oil misters, soy, and non-alcohol no sugar flavorings.

This book is neither sponsored by nor endorsed by any organization. It serves the function of press. It gives information. Many men and women weigh and measure food as part of a personal plan of recovery from problem eating. Many recovering individuals DO NOT weigh and measure food. There are many strong feelings about it. The editors take no position on weighing and measuring or the sample plans of eating illustrated.

The thoughts in this reader are not intended to diagnose or treat or cure any illness and do not constitute medical advice. We are not engaged in rendering medical, nutritional, dietetic or other professional information. If medical, nutritional, or diatetic advice or other expert advice is required, the services of a competent professional person should be sought. The best safeguard against either compulsive eating or compulsive dieting is an active participation in the Twelve Step Programs of Recovery. We remember that no Twelve Step Program member plays Doctor.

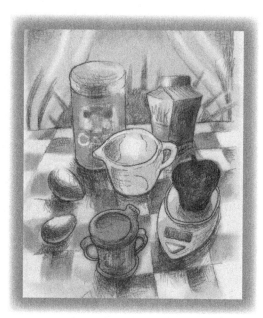

CHAPTER 1
Ways to Use This Book

WAYS YOU MAY USE THIS COOKBOOK

1. You may use this cookbook in several ways. You may use it to see *Sample Plans of Eating*. There are seven Sample Plans of Eating illustrated – some with starches and grains and some with no starches or grains. See websites to obtain plans of eating supported by non-profit overeating and food addiction groups..

2. You may use it for *300 Recipes - No Sugar-Wheat-Flour - Everything Weighed and Measured, With and Without Starches and Grains.*

3. You may use it to learn about *The 'Science & Spirit' of Meals vs Pounce or Grazing* written by a Twelve Step Recovery member.

4. You may use it to hear one contributor's take on *The Benefits & Eating with Safety & Security.*

5. You may read *To Weigh & Measure or To Not Weigh & Measure* and learn about *The Phenomenon of Weighing & Measuring.*

6. You may use it as a way to "Get Started" with sample plans of eating and recipes, either on your own, or with someone who is willing to support you with letting go of compulsive eating. Anyone can weigh and measure any food at any time, from any recipe, meal combination, or plan of eating.

7. You may use it to learn about *People & Groups* who support letting go of compulsive eating, to get phone numbers to attend free phone meetings, phone someone, or work with someone to be your phone buddy or sponsor.

8. You may use it to see illustrations from – *Cups & Scales – Weighing & Measuring Food & Emotions.* See some of *The Attitudes of the Cups & Scales.* It is not using cups and scales that makes my recovery. It is my perspective toward food and life that helps make life manageable and joyous. When I am at peace with my food and my emotions, I can be at peace with others.

TO WEIGH & MEASURE OR TO NOT WEIGH & MEASURE?

Over the years a practice has grown up where many people weigh and measure their food as part of a personal plan of eating and recovery from compulsive overeating, food addiction, anorexia, bulimia, emotional eating and other eating disorders. The weighing and measuring gives a physical as much as a spiritual boundary for the eating. It offers perspective, pause, and thought. Many consider it helpful in eating right. Eating right to many is a spiritual condition. Many people weigh and measure to see the perspective it gives them. They incorporate the experience into their lives. Many may not weigh and measure at all times or in all places. They may use the practice at various times.

There are many women and men recovering who DO NOT weigh and measure their food. The editors take no position on weighing and measuring food. There are many strong feelings about it. This book is neither endorsed by nor sponsored by any organization.

WHO WEIGHS & MEASURES?
WHERE YOU CAN FIND SUPPORT
WHETHER YOU WEIGH & MEASURE OR NOT

There are many groups that recommend and support the practice. There are people and groups that don't support the practice. You may find support to let go of compulsive eating in many groups. This includes people in *Compulsive Overeaters Anonymous-HOW; Cups & Scales Forum; Food Addicts Anonymous; Food Addicts: The Body Knows Online Discussion Group; Greysheeter's Anonymous; Overeaters Anonymous, regular OA meetings & OA H.O.W. and 90-Day meetings; and Recovery from Food Addiction.* Contacts are willing to be your phone buddy or to sponsor you. In this book you get access to free phone meeting numbers, websites, and email addresses to contact people and groups. For resources and links to these people and groups see Chapter 9.

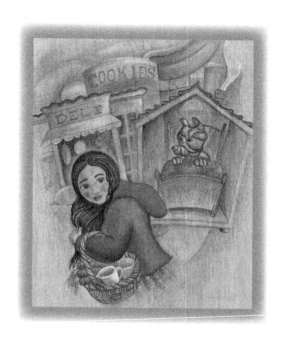

CHAPTER 2
Benefits ~
I Eat with Safety & Security

"A Cups & Scales Compact"

From Anonymous

I use cups and scales to eat with safety and security for my better ordering and preservation and to further my understanding.

1. I start by eating. I have the right to eat. I have never lost the right to eat. I don't diet, restrict, use diet pills or other diet remedies, restrict or skip meals. Another meal is coming.

2. I shop and buy the right foods. I plan my meals and buy the right foods. This gives me safety and security knowing the right food is near me. It is ready to use.

3. I get rid of any trigger foods in the house. I don't keep them around. I don't buy them, pretending they are for others, then to eat them myself. If trigger foods come into the house, brought in by me, I throw them out as quickly as I am able.

4. If foods that trigger me have to be in the house for others, I don't handle them. I ask others to keep trigger foods in a separate cupboard where I don't go.

5. I have safety and security in knowing another meal is coming. I know where I will get it, how it will be made, and what will be in it, food choices, ingredients, and portions.

6. Because I know where I will get my food and what will be in it, I have comfort. I can make it from city block to city block and road to road without going into the carbohydrate stores or fast food stores. I don't have to eat other people's food. I have my own.

7. I choose a plan of eating for the day. I use cups & scales to eat with safety and security for my better ordering and preservation. This gives me clarity, ease of conscience, freedom to eat, and protection from encroaching food fears, massive amounts of food, or the wrong foods.

8. Weighing and measuring and eating my measured meals gives me nutrition, right brain functioning, and energy balance.

9. I think in terms of weighed and measured amounts. The weighing and measuring gives me a physical as much as a spiritual boundary for my eating. When possible I prepare my own food, measuring ingredients and portions. When cups and scales are not available to me or I plan to eat food out or prepared by others, I find out about ingredients, weights and measures, and food preparation before choosing a food or eating a food. I choose weighed and measured amounts. I choose foods with ingredients and portions I would use when I am preparing my own food at home.

10. I care for my own food. I take responsibility for food choices, how many meals I will have and frequency of meals. I get the right ingredients, weigh and measure ingredients, and weigh and measure my portions. I remember to eat. I eat my prepared food.

A Cups & Scales Compact is inspired *The Mayflower Compact* which I recently read at an exhibit. *The Mayflower Compact* is a piece of living history saying how the people on landing in a new land agree to create a self-government for better ordering and preservation. *A Cups & Scales Compact* explains how I make a compact for my better ordering and preservation. – *Contributor's Note.*

Benefits of Eating with Safety & Security

- I Cook & Eat With Happiness
- I Cook & Eat Without Remorse
- I Care for My Own Food
- I Get Nutrition
- I Get Peace of Mind on a Plate

Because I Care For My Own Food?

- I am safe
- I have never lost the right to eat
- I have another meal coming
- I have the comfort of knowing where I will get my next meal
- I have the safety, security & comfort of knowing what will be in it
- I have no reason for guilt. I am safe
- I use cups and scales for my better ordering and preservation
- I get clarity and understanding
- I benefit from the science and spirit of meals

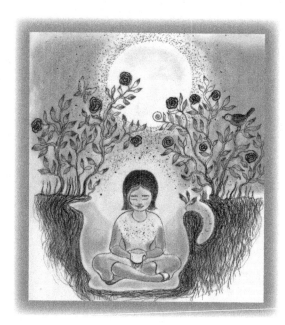

CHAPTER 3
Sample Plans of Eating

WHERE CAN I FIND SAMPLE PLANS OF EATING?

SAMPLE PLANS OF EATING: SAMPLE PLANS 1-7

The Plans of Eating shown here are for educational illustration purposes only. They indicate:

1) what food groups you might include,
2) what food groups might be in a meal,
3) what you might choose for a serving,
4) the number of servings in a food group in a recipe, and
5) the frequency of meals you might choose.

Recipes have weighed and measured amounts.

This cookbook does not endorse or recommend any specific plan of eating. People with specific dietary needs, especially pregnant women and men, and those who are vegans or vegetarians, lactose intolerant, or have specific food allergies, need to construct your individual personal plan of eating with a health professional. Each person needs to consult their health practitioner.

We remember that no Twelve Step Program member plays Doctor. The thoughts in this reader are not intended to diagnose or treat or cure any illness and do not constitute medical advice. We are not engaged in rendering medical, nutritional, dietetic or other professional information. If medical, nutritional, or diatetic advice or other expert advice is required, the services of a competent professional person should be sought. The best safeguard against either compulsive eating or compulsive dieting is an active participation in the Twelve Step Programs of Recovery.

Seven sample plans of eating are illustrated - plans with one fruit to four fruits per day, and plans with and without starches and grains. Use the recipes in this book separately or in combination with a plan of eating.

See non-profit overeating and food addiction group websites listed here where you may obtain the plans of eating they support.

"Facing Plan of Eating Choices with My Healthcare Practitioner & A Sponsor"
An Essay by Anonymous

Choosing a Plan of Eating requires spiritual recovery, honesty, and consideration. What are my purposes? Choosing a personal plan should be done in concert with another person, preferably with both a health care practitioner and a sponsor.

It is alright to talk to my doctor about weight loss. I am not anti-doctor or against plans of eating. However, there is a fact – I have abused compulsive dieting. My life-enhancing decision to let go of compulsive dieting needs to be foremost in my communication with my doctor and in choosing a plan of eating. My doctor can work with me for my physical and mental health by having complete information about me. I let my doctor know my background, my experience, my susceptibilities

Like the recovering alcoholic, some of us compulsive eaters and compulsive dieters have used dieting methods and schemes.

I find the ideas expressed in the *A.A. Conference Approved Statement on Drug Use* helpful (Alcoholics Anonymous, 1995). To paraphrase it and apply it to use of a plan of eating – I am aware of the misuse of dieting methods and schemes. At the same time, just as it would be wrong to enable or support anyone to become re-addicted to compulsive dieting methods or schemes, it would be wrong to deprive anyone of a plan of eating which can be used as a tool to alleviate disabling eating problems. I find these suggestions helpful to me.

1. I will remember that as a person recovering from compulsive dieting and compulsive eating my automatic response will be to turn to the quick fix for uncomfortable feelings. I will look for non-quick-fix solutions for the aches and discomforts of everyday living. I will not consider a plan of eating a quick fix.

2. I will remember that the best safeguard against a compulsive dieting relapse or a compulsive eating relapse is an active participation in the Twelve Step Programs of Recovery.

3. I remember that no Twelve Step Program member plays Doctor. Consult your physician for medical advice.

4. I am completely honest with myself and my physician regarding my thinking on use of a plan of eating. Such honesty is important to me and my doctor.

5. I consult a physician with experience, knowledge of my medical history, and an awareness of the problems associated with compulsive dieting and compulsive eating.

6. I inform the physician at once if I experience side effects from a food or a plan of eating.

7. I communicate with my health professional on a regular basis.

I Can Make a Personal Plan of Eating

I can construct a personal plan of eating with my health professional. Then I can construct meals using the recipes here. Recipes here have weighed and measured amounts to a serving.

1. I get to know myself.

2. I let go of magical thinking about any plan of eating I might be considering.

3. My life-enhancing decision to let go of compulsive dieting is foremost in choosing a plan of eating.

4. I am free to talk about choices in plans of eating to my health care professional and sponsor.

5. I can talk to others about their experiences with any personal plan of eating they may follow. Yet I know I am an individual.

6. I can change the personal plan of eating I have chosen to another one at any time. I stay in touch with myself and communicate with my health professional and my sponsor on a regular basis.

Weighing & Measuring ~ A Practice Independent From Choosing & Working Within A Plan of Eating

Choosing a plan of eating needs to be done with consideration. It may take time to talk to a healthcare practitioner, think about it, talk to others, talk to a sponsor. Yet do not hesitate. It is worth eating regular planned meals.

Weighing and measuring can be done at anytime. Anyone can weigh and measure any food at any time, from any recipe, meal combination, or plan of eating. Weighing and measuring is an issue independent from choosing and working within a plan of eating.

Sample Plans Of Eating No Sugar - Wheat - Flour

WITH STARCH/GRAINS

PLAN 1:

    FOUR FRUITS PER DAY
    WITH STARCH/GRAINS
    SUITABLE FOR THREE MEALS A DAY (3)
    OR SIX HALF MEALS PER DAY (6)
    WITH AFTER DINNER/BEDTIME METABOLIC

BREAKFAST

» 2 ozs. protein serving = 2 ozs. protein (weighed)
» or 1 egg, or 1 ozs protein and 1/2 oz hard cheese
» 1 starch/grain serving = 1/2 cup cooked
   or 1 oz. (dry weighed uncooked)
» 1 fruit serving = 6 ozs fruit
» 1 cup milk or milk substitute

LUNCH

» 3 ozs. protein serving = 3 ozs. protein (weighed)
» 1 starch/grain serving = 1/2 cup (cooked)
   or 1 oz. (dry weighed uncooked)
» 1 fruit serving = 6 ozs. fruit
» 3 vegetable servings = 1 ½ cups or
   12 ozs. vegetable (weighed)
» fat = 2 tsps oil or fat (10-12 grams fat at meal)

DINNER

» 3 ozs. protein serving = 3 ozs. protein (weighed)
» or same options as lunch,
» 1 starch/grain serving = 1/2 cup (cooked)
   or 1 oz. (dry weighed uncooked)
» 1 fruit serving = 6 ozs. Fruit
» 3 vegetable servings = 1 ½ cups
   or 12 ozs. veg. (weighed)
» fat = 2 tsps oil or fat(10-12 grams fat at meal)

BEDTIME/AFTER DINNER METABOLIC

» 1 starch/grain serving = 1/2 cup cooked
» 1 fruit serving = 6 ozs. Fruit
» 1 cup milk or milk substitute

(Plan 1: fat servings = 20-24 grams fat total day =
1 tablespoon & 1 teaspoon = 4 tsps. day)

PLAN 2:

    FOUR FRUITS PER DAY
    WITH STARCH/GRAINS
    SUITABLE FOR THREE MEALS A DAY (3)
    OR SIX HALF MEALS PER DAY (6)
    WITH AFTER DINNER/BEDTIME METABOLIC

BREAKFAST

» 2 starch/grain serving = 1/2 cup x 2 = 1 cup
   cooked or 2 oz. grain (dry weighed uncooked)
» 1 fruit serving = 6 ozs. fruit
» 1 cup milk or milk substitute

LUNCH

» 2 ozs. protein serving = 2 ozs. protein (weighed)
» or 2 eggs, or 2 ozs protein and 1 oz hard cheese
» 2 starch/grain servings = 1/2 cup x 2 = 1 cup
   cooked or 2 oz. (dry weighed uncooked)
» 1 fruit serving = 6 ozs. fruit
» 3 vegetable servings = 1 ½ cups or
   12 ozs. vegetable (weighed)
» fat serving = 2 tsps oil or fat (10-
   12 grams fat at meal)

DINNER

» 2 ozs. protein serving = 2 ozs protein (weighed)
» or same options as lunch
» 2 starch/grain servings = 1/2 cup x 2 = 1 cup
   cooked or 2 ozs. (dry weighed uncooked)
» 3 vegetable servings = 1 ½ cups or
   12 ozs. vegetable (weighed)
» fat = 2 tsps oil or fat (10-12 grams fat at meal)

BEDTIME/AFTER DINNER METABOLIC

» 2 starch/grain serving = 1/2
   cup x 2 = 1 cup cooked
» 1 fruit serving = 6 ozs. fruit

(Plan 2: fat servings = 20-24 grams fat total day =
1 tablespoon & 1 teaspoon = 4 tsps. day)

Sample Plans Of Eating No Sugar - Wheat - Flour

WITH STARCH/GRAINS

PLAN 3:

THREE FRUITS PER DAY
WITH STARCH/GRAINS
SUITABLE FOR THREE MEALS A DAY (3)
OR SIX HALF-MEALS PER DAY (6)

BREAKFAST
» 2 ozs. protein serving = 2 ozs protein (weighed)
» or 1 egg, or 1 ozs. hard cheese
» 2 starch/grain servings = 1/2 cup x 2 = 1 cup
cooked or 2 ozs. (dry weighed uncooked)
» 1 fruit serving = 6 ozs. fruit
» 2 cups milk or milk substitute

LUNCH
» 4 ozs. protein serving = 4 ozs. protein (weighed)
or 2 eggs, or 2 ozs protein and 1 oz hard cheese
, or 2 ozs. protein (weighed) & 1 cup milk,
» or 2 ozs. protein (weighed) and 1 egg,
» or 1 ozs. hard cheese (weighed) and 1 egg
or 1 ozs. hard cheese and 1 cup milk
» 2 starch/grain servings = 1/2 cup x 2 = 1 cup
cooked or 2 ozs. (dry weighed uncooked)
» 1 fruit serving = 6 ozs. fruit
» 2 vegetable servings = 1 cup or 8 ozs. (weighed)
» fat servings = 2 tsps. oil or fat (10-
12 grams fat at meal)

DINNER
» 4 ozs. protein serving = 4 ozs. protein (weighed)
» or same options as lunch
» 2 starch/grain servings = 1/2 cup x 2 = 1 cup
cooked or 2 ozs. (dry weighed uncooked)
» 1 fruit serving = 6 ozs. fruit
» 3 vegetable servings = 1 ½ cups or
12 ozs. vegetable (weighed)
» fat servings = 2 tsps oil or fat (10-
12 grams fat at meal)

(Plan 3: fat servings = 20-24 grams fat total day =
1 tablespoon & 1 teaspoon = 4 tsps. day)

PLAN 4:

TWO FRUITS PER DAY
WITH STARCH/GRAINS
SUITABLE FOR THREE MEALS A DAY (3)
OR SIX HALF MEALS PER DAY (6)
WITH AFTER DINNER/BEDTIME METABOLIC

BREAKFAST
» 4 ozs. protein serving = 4 ozs protein (weighed)
» or 2 eggs, or 2 ozs protein and 1 oz hard cheese
» 1 starch/grain serving = 1/2 cup cooked
or 1 oz. (dry weighed uncooked)
» 1 fruit serving = 6 ozs. fruit
» 1 cup milk or milk substitute

LUNCH
» 4 ozs. protein serving = 4 ozs. protein (weighed)
» or 2 eggs, or 2 ozs protein and 1 oz hard cheese
» 4 vegetable servings = 1/2 cup x 4 =
2 cups or 16 ozs. vegetable (weighed)
» fat serving = 3 tsps = 1 tbs oil or fat
(14-16 grams fat at meal)

DINNER
» 4 ozs. protein serving = 4 ozs protein (weighed)
» or same options as lunch,
» 4 vegetable servings = 1/2 cup x 4 =
2 cups or 16 ozs. vegetable (weighed)
» fat serving = 3 tsps = 1 tbs oil or fat
(14-16 grams fat at meal)

BEDTIME/AFTER DINNER METABOLIC
» 1 fruit serving = 6 ozs. fruit
» 1 cup milk or milk substitute

(Plan 4: fat servings = 28-32 grams fat total day =
2 tablespoons = 6 teaspoons day)

Sample Plans Of Eating No Sugar - Wheat - Flour

WITH STARCH/GRAINS

PLAN 5:

TWO FRUITS PER DAY WITH
STARCH/GRAINS
SUITABLE FOR THREE MEALS A DAY (3)
OR SIX HALF MEALS PER DAY (6)
WITH AFTER DINNER/
BEDTIME METABOLIC

BREAKFAST

» 4 ozs. protein serving = 4 ozs. protein (weighed)
» or 2 eggs, or 2 ozs protein and 1 oz hard cheese
» 1 cup starch/grain (cooked) or 2
  oz. (dry weighed uncooked)
» 1 fruit serving = 6 ozs fruit
» 1 cup milk or milk substitute

LUNCH

» 4 ozs. protein serving = 4 ozs. protein (weighed)
» 3 vegetable servings = 1 ½ cups
  or 12 ozs. veg. (weighed)
» ½ fat serving = 1 ½ tsps oil or fat
» (7-8 grams fat at meal)

DINNER

» 4 ozs. protein serving = 4 ozs. protein (weighed)
» or same options as lunch,
» 1 cup starch/grain (cooked) or 2
  ozs. (dry weighed uncooked)
» 3 vegetable servings = 1 ½ cups
  or 12 ozs. veg. (weighed)
» ½ fat serving = 1 ½ tsps oil or fat
» (7-8 grams fat at meal)

BEDTIME/AFTER DINNER METABOLIC

» 1 fruit serving = 6 ozs. Fruit
» 1 cup milk or milk substitute

(Plan 5: fat = 14-16 grams fat total day =
1 tablespoon = 3 tsps. day)

PLAN 6:

TWO FRUITS PER DAY WITH
STARCH/GRAINS
SUITABLE FOR THREE MEALS A DAY (3)
OR SIX HALF MEALS PER DAY (6)
WITH AFTER DINNER/
BEDTIME METABOLIC

BREAKFAST

» 2 ozs. protein serving = 2 ozs. protein (weighed)
» or 1 egg, or 1 ozs protein and 1/2 oz hard cheese
» 1 cup starch/grain (cooked) or 2
  oz. (dry weighed uncooked)
» 1 fruit serving = 6 ozs fruit
» 1 cup milk or milk substitute

LUNCH

» 4 ozs. protein serving = 4 ozs. protein (weighed)
» 1 cup starch/grain (cooked) or 2
  ozs (dry weighed uncooked)
» 3 vegetable servings = 1 ½ cups
  or 12 ozs. veg. (weighed)
» ½ fat serving = 1 ½ tsps. oil or fat
» (7-8 grams fat at meal)

DINNER

» 4 ozs. protein serving = 4 ozs. protein (weighed)
» or same options as lunch,
» 1 cup starch/grain (cooked) or 2
  ozs. (dry weighed uncooked)
» 3 vegetable servings = 1 ½ cups
  or 12 ozs. veg. (weighed)
» ½ fat servings = 1 ½ tsps. oil or fat
» (7-8 grams fat at meal)

BEDTIME/AFTER DINNER METABOLIC

» 1 fruit serving = 6 ozs. Fruit
» 1 cup milk or milk substitute

(Plan 6: fat = 14-16 grams fat total day =
1 tablespoon = 3 tsps. day)

Sample Plans Of Eating No Sugar - Wheat - Flour

WITHOUT STARCH/GRAINS

PLAN 7:

ONE FRUIT PER DAY
NO STARCH/GRAINS
SUITABLE FOR THREE MEALS A DAY (3)
OR SIX HALF MEALS PER DAY (6)

BREAKFAST
» 4 ozs. protein serving = 4 ozs. protein (weighed)
   or 2 eggs, or 2 ozs protein and 1oz hard cheese
   or 2 ozs. protein (weighed) & 1 cup milk
» 1 fruit serving = 6 ozs fruit

LUNCH
» 4 ozs. protein serving = 4 ozs. protein (weighed)
   or 2 eggs, or 2 ozs protein and 1oz hard cheese
   or 2 ozs. protein (weighed) & 1 cup milk
» 1 cup cooked vegetables =8 ozs. cooked
» vegetable (weighed measure)
» 2 cups raw vegetables = 16 ozs.
   raw egetable (weighed)
» 1 ½ tsp oil (7-8 grams fat at meal)

DINNER
» 4 ozs. protein serving = 4 ozs. protein (weighed)
» or same options as lunch
» 1 cup cooked vegetable = 1 cups or
   8 ozs. vegetable (weighed)
» 1 cup cooked vegetables = 1 cup = 8 ozs. cooked
» 2 cups raw vegetables = 16 ozs.
   raw egetable (weighed)
» 1 ½ tsp oil (7-8 grams fat at meal)

(Plan 7: fat = 14-16 grams fat total day =
1 tablespoon = 3 tsps.

WHAT ARE THE PLANS OF EATING SUPPORTED BY NON-PROFIT OVEREATING & FOOD ADDICTION GROUPS?

Here is a brief list of groups and websites where you may obtain plans of eating non-profit overeating and food addiction groups support. The list also indicates whether the group supports weighing and measuring and whether it suggests or requires the practice.

Chapter 9 gives more information on free phone meeting numbers, websites, face-to-face meetings, and email addresses to contact people. Contacts are willing

to be your phone buddy or to sponsor you.

CEA-HOW (Compulsive Overeaters Anonymous-HOW) – Requires Weighing & Measuring

http://www.ceahow.org/
gso@ceahow
- Weighing & Measuring is required.
- There is a required plan of eating. It includes fruit, dairy, protein and vegetables. The CEA-HOW plan of eating is available from "Achieving Balance Cookbook" at the website: http://www.ceahow.org/?q=node/11

Cups & Scales Online Forum – Discusses Weighing & Measuring

Cupsandscales-subscribe@yahoogroups.com
- Weighing & Measuring may be freely discussed in the forum. The moderators take no position on it. It may be freely discussed. There are many strong feelings about it.
- There is no suggested or endorsed plan of eating required.
- Cups & Scales takes its name from the book *Cups & Scales, Weighing & Measuring Food & Emotions* by Anonymous Twelve Step Recovery Members.
  Cups & Scales Everything Weighed & Measured Cookbook – 7 Sample Plans of Eating - 300 Recipes - No Sugar, Wheat, Flour - With & Without Starches & Grains. These books are recommended literature.

Food Addicts Anonymous (FAA) — Recommends Weighing & Measuring

http://www.foodaddictsanonymous.org/meetings-events
561-967-3871

- Weighing & Measuring is recommended.
- There is a recommended FAA plan of eating. It includes fruit, dairy, protein, vegetables, and starches and grains. People follow a food plan devoid of all addictive substances, including sugar, flour and wheat in all their forms. These substances also include fats and any other high-carbohydrate, refined, processed foods that cause problems individually.
- The FAA recommended plan of eating is found on the website: http://www. foodaddictsanonymous.org/faa-food-plan.

Food Addiction: The Body Knows — Suggests Weighing & Measuring

http://www.kaysheppard.com/
kshepp825@aol.com
321-727-8040
thebodyknows-subscribe@yahoogroups.com

- Weighing & Measuring is suggested.
- There is a suggested plan of eating. It includes fruit, dairy, protein, vegetables, and starches and grains. People follow a food plan devoid of all addictive substances, including sugar, flour and wheat in all their forms. These substances also include fats and any other high-carbohydrate, refined, processed foods that cause problems individually. is similar to the plan of eating recommended in Food Addicts Anonymous. It includes an additional serving of starch and grain at lunch. The plan of eating recommends no caffein, no sweeteners and weighed and measured servings.
- The FA: TBN recommended plan of eating is found on the website: http://www.kaysheppard.com.

Recovery From Food Addiction (RFA) – Suggests Weighing & Measuring

Recoveryfromfoodaddiction-subscribe@yahoogroups.com
- Weighing & Measuring is recommended.
- There is a suggested plan of eating. It includes fruit, dairy, protein, vegetables, and starches and grains. People follow a food plan devoid of all addictive substances, including sugar, flour and wheat in all their forms. These substances also include fats and any other high-carbohydrate, refined, processed foods that cause problems individually. The suggested plan of eating is similar to the plan of eating recommended in Food Addicts Anonymous. It includes an additional serving of starch and grain at lunch. The plan of eating recommends no caffein, no sweeteners and weighed and measured servings.
- The RFA recommended plan of eating is found on the website: http://www.kaysheppard.com.

Greysheeters Anonymous (GSA) – Requires Weighing & Measuring

http://www.greysheet.org/cms/
uscontacts@greysheet.org
phonelist@greysheet.org
- Weighing & Measuring from The Greysheet Food Plan is required.
- There is a required plan of eating. The Greysheet Food Plan comes with a Sponsor. The Greysheet Food Plan was originally offered for suggestion by Overeater's Anonymous Inc. in the 1960's, a very low carb, high protein food plan, no grains, no breads, flour products, only products that list sugar at least fifth on the label, and quantities suggested in weighed and measured amounts.

Overeaters Anonymous Inc. — Takes No Position on Weighing & Measuring
Specific Meetings Support Weighing & Measuring

http://www.oa.org
505-891-2664

- Overeaters Anonymous neither endorses nor supports any specific plan of eating. There is no sponsored or endorsed plan of eating. The OA pamphlet *"The Dignity of Choice"* explains different plans of eating and recommends that an individual work with their nutritionist or healthcare practitioner in choosing a plan of eating as part of a personal plan of recovery (*The Dignity of Choice,* Overeaters Anonymous, 1972).

- While the Overeaters Anonymous Inc. organization takes no position on weighing and measuring, specific meetings within OA, such as O.A. H.O.W. and 90-Day meetings, support weighing and measuring. These specific meetings state that support in their descriptions on the OA website, www.oa.org:

OA H.O.W. Program — Requires Weighing & Measuring

- Weighing & Measuring is required.
- We do not write our own food plan. We use a food plan given to us by a doctor, nutritionist or dietician. We discuss it with our sponsor. We do not pick one that allows any of our binge foods. If some food on our plan becomes a problem, we avoid it.

"H.O.W. is a movement within Overeaters Anonymous whose basic principle is that abstinence is the only means to freedom from compulsive overeating and the beginning of a spiritual life. We believe that the discipline of weighing and measuring, of telephoning your sponsor at a particular time, of attending meetings and making phone calls; all lead to a life based on the Universal Discipline, which is accord rather than discord even with many things going on around us. We eat weighed and measured meals with nothing in between except sugar free beverages and sugar free gum.

- Food is written down, called in to our sponsor and committed, so that we can get on with our recovery and out of the food.
- We do not skip meals, switch meals or combine meals. We do not deviate or manipulate our food plan in any way. If we need to change our committed food during the day, we call a sponsor.
- We weigh and measure all our portions so that there is no guess work. We do not measure by eye. We use a measuring cup, spoon, and a scale.

- We weigh ourselves once a month until we reach goal weight and once a week on maintenance.
- Unless advised otherwise by your doctor, we take a multi-vitamin and drink 64 oz. of water a day.
- We do not drink alcohol.
- We do not use foods containing sugar, except if sugar is listed 5th or beyond on the ingredients label (Overeaters Anonymous Inc, 2010, http://www.oa.org)."

90-DAY Program - Suggests Weighing & Measuring

- Weighing & Measuring is recommended.
- Overeaters Anonymous neither endorses nor supports any specific plan of eating. There is no sponsored or endorsed "90-Day" OA plan of eating. The OA pamphlet "Dignity of Choice" explains different plans of eating and recommends that an individual work with their nutritionist or healthcare practitioner in choosing a plan of eating as part of a personal plan of recovery.
- 90-Day Meetings give help to people who want a structured approach, including weighing and measuring, calling a Sponsor daily, making three outreach calls daily, and 90 days abstinence to share on phone meetings
(Overeaters Anonymous Inc, 2010, http://www.oa.org)."

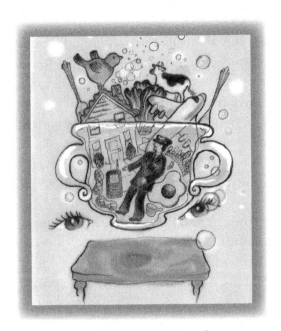

CHAPTER 4
Frequencies of Meals

"How Many Meals a Day?

So I don't Get Hungry?

For Metabolism?

For Special Needs & Purposes?

So I don't Pick Up Trigger Foods?"

An Essay by Anonymous

The number of times I need to eat a meal depends on several things – hunger, metabolic needs, and special needs and purposes.

These factors can be discussed with my healthcare practitioner and a sponsor in a Twelve Step Recovery Program.

Here are some possible special needs and accommodations to be talked about with my healthcare practitioner and a sponsor in a Twelve Step Recovery Program.

1. I have to get to know myself. If I get hungry between meals (after eliminating sugar and flour from my diet), maybe I need to eat more frequently. Maybe I need to have less time between meals. Maybe I need to eat more slowly and take extra time to eat the meal. Maybe I will have 6 half meals a day, eating every 3-4 hours, instead of three meals a day, eating 4.5-5 hours apart.

2. If I am trying to give up sugar and flour from my diet, maybe I need to eat a diet without sugar and flour, with more frequent meals – more than 3 meals a day – so I don't get hungry between meals, and have enough real food, and CAN give up sugar and flour. Maybe I will have 6 half meals a day, eating every 3-4 hours, instead of three meals a day.

3. If I am hyperglycemic or diabetic, what does my health practitioner recommend with my sugar levels? Maybe they will recommend eating smaller meals, more frequently. I will choose to have 6 half meals a day, eating every 3-4 hours, instead of three meals a day.

Regular scheduling of meals ensures I am safe and secure. I know another meal is coming. I can get on with other activities – because I know another meal is coming and when it is scheduled. I do not need to respond to food availability cues when food may be constantly available. Hunger will appear around the time of the scheduled meal. My hunger cues from my brain will be accustomed to expect another meal within a certain time frame.

Special needs and accommodations can be talked about with my healthcare practitioner and a sponsor in a Twelve Step Recovery Program. I have freedom to choose the number and frequency of my meals.

What Are Adjustable Frequencies of Meals?

Here are some timeframes for adjustable frequencies of meals.
The Sample Plans of Eating show they are suitable for adjustable frequencies of meals.

Three Meals A Day

Suitable for Six Half Meals A Day — Plus Bedtime Metabolic

With three meals a day, we eat every 4.5 to 5 hours.

Breakfast	Lunch	Dinner	Bedtime/Metabolic
Starting at:			
7:00 A.M. .	11:30 - 12:00	5:00 - 6:00	7:00-8:00 or 8:00-9:00 P.M.
8:00 A.M..	12:30 - 1:00 .	6:00 - 7:00	8:00 - 9:00 or 9:00 -10:00 P.M.
9:00 A.M.	1:30 - 2:00	7:00 - 8:00	9:00-10:00 - 10:00-11:00 P.M.-
10:00 A.M.	2:30 - 3:00	8:00 - 9:00	10:30-11:00 or 11:30-12:30 P.M.
11:00 A.M.	3:30 - 4:00	10:00 - 11:00	12:00-1:00 or 12:30-1:30 A.M.

With six meals a day, we eat every 2.5 to 4 hours

Breakfast		Lunch		Dinner		Bedtime/Metabolic
Starting at:						
7:00 A.M.	9:30	12:00	2:30	5:00	7:30	8:00-9:00 or 9:00-10:00 P.M.
8:00 A.M.	10:30	1:00	3:30	6:00	8:30	9:00-10:00 or 10:00-11:00 P.M.
9:00 A.M.	11:30	2:00	4:30	7:00	9:30	10:00-11:00 or 11:00-12:00 P.M.

An after dinner-before bedtime metabolic is in place on some of the Sample Plans of Eating. It helps to prevent a drop in blood sugar over many hours, to satisfy hunger 2-4 hours after dinner, and to prevent nighttime hunger and eating.

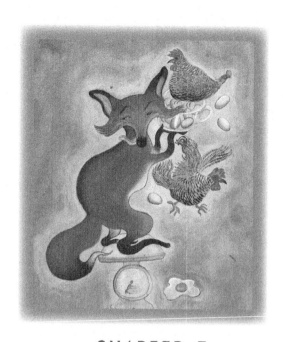

CHAPTER 5
"The 'Science & Spirit' of Meals vs. Pounce or Grazing"

WHAT DO I GET FROM MEALS: AN ESSAY BY ANONYMOUS

MY DEEP SYSTEM – MY BIOLOGY & CHEMISTRY

Glucose – glycolysis – cellular respiration. Glucose is necessary for glycolysis. Glycolysis allows cellular respiration - the very biological process whereby energy is created to sustain my life. Opportunity, food availability, the desire to eat, the taste to eat, the taste for sweetness built into my taste buds – all these are part of the natural history, the biological history, the backdrop, that has shaped my being here today. They are part of my deep system (*Biology: Life on Earth with Physiology*, 2010).

In my culture, food is available 24/7. It is possible to find sweetness, either sucrose or other forms of sugar 24/7. At an earlier time in human history, the opportunity to eat and the availability of food was far less.

Within my culture I could eat all the time or gravitate toward the taste for sweetness all the time. The conditions of my life are different from that of my ancestors. Yet the need to find accommodations to survive are the same. Let's look at *"The Science & Spirit of Meals."*

What is the Difference between Grazing & Pounce & Eating a Meal?

"Creation gave us instincts for a purpose," it says in the *Alcoholics Anonymous Twelve Steps & Twelve Traditions* (AA, *Twelve Steps & Twelve Traditions*, 1953).

In the "wild," animals graze or pounce.

Undomesticated "wild" mammals, like wolfs, coyotes, cheetahs hunt and pounce. So do amphibians, insects and fish. In the moment of impact, hunting becomes devouring. Devouring insures quick energy intake and survival. Food may not be available for long. Another animal may chase the first away from the food source; the coyote may be chased away by the wolf, so eating quickly becomes doubly important.

Slow-chewing domesticated mammals "graze." Cows, goats and sheep, with several stomachs, graze on grasses, digest it in slow-chewing, and move on to greener pastures, where the grass hasn't been grazed and isn't as short.

Grazing and pouncing has its place. It is built-in instinct. It serves a purpose for each animal in its habitat.

The Social Instinct — Necessary for Survival

For us humans, meals serve another purpose – a social instinct. Not merely eating together, but hunting together, and the delay of food consumption, after the gathering or hunt, so food may be shared, emerges from cooperation and fosters cooperation and intelligence. Planning.

Traditionally, the meal, the sharing of food after the hunt, has meant tribe survival. There would be severe sanctions if a single member stole or hoarded or pounced on food, excluding others (*Mutual Aid*, Kropotkin).

The development of law and order by people has grown out of the social instinct – the need for those in the group to survive, and has served the needs of both the individual and the community. Delay of gratification is important. It means other considerations besides immediate gratification come into play. Human communities have grown by cooperating, creating standards of behavior and laws around many things including eating, delay and sharing. The standards and traditions developed around food consumption have served the social instinct.

MEAL-TAKING SHOWS THE NEEDED COMMON BOND

THE ECONOMIC BACKGROUND OF FOOD EARNING

FOOD IS PRECIOUS

In Charles Dickens' English tale, "*A Christmas Carol*", the breadwinner, Mr. Jacob Marley, asks the boss, Mr. Ebenezer Scrooge, permission to leave work early so he can pick up the Christmas goose to rush home to be with the family he works so hard to feed.

Meal-taking shows the common bond.

In the French novel, *Germinale*, by Emile Zola a coal mining family in 19th Century France struggles to earn food money by going to work in the coal mines. When there is not enough work or money for food, the old grandfather who no longer works and the infant starve. The working adults get the little food there is.

In the Danish tale, "*The Little Match Girl*", by Hans Christian Anderson, a poor girl alone, on the streets, freezing, mindless with hunger, lights the last of her three matches and has an emblazoned vision of a holiday feast, before she drops in the snow. She is on the outside looking in. People eating together are provided for.

Stories in our literature remind us about our need for food and community. Food is precious. A valued commodity, it is worked for; it is paid for with hard labor and well-earned money; people pay good money for food; they value precious food.

CHANGES IN THE PATTERN OF MEAL-TAKING

The pattern of meal-taking has changed in the last 100 years. Conditions have made it possible for there to be more energy available to humans from high caloric foods, more food, and less starvation in many parts of the world. Cooperation has made it possible for specialized groups of people or the agri-business industries to grow the food for the many. With food available at stores 24/7, and individuals earning individual wages, individuals can buy their own food, anytime. The changes or freedoms afforded by modern food supply, availability, and convenience are these:

- I can eat anytime.
- With food preservatives I can eat from vending machines.
- Food doesn't have to be fresh.
- Food can be packaged with preservatives in cellophane.
- Food doesn't have to be food. It can be chemical soup.
- With fast food restaurants, I can eat food frozen thousands of miles away, shipped thousands of miles, unthawed, and cooked days or months after leaving the source where it was grown or packaged. .
- I can drive through a fast food restaurant and don't have to sit down.
- I can grab food on the run. I don't have to eat with others.
- The fast food imperative says 'I must be in a rush. Why else would the convenience store or fast food restaurant be here?'
- I can snack anytime I want.
- I can eat 24/7.
- I have 24/7 exposure to food.
- I can isolate. No one else has to know what I am eating.

The individual freedoms offered by the food industry marketplace can alter many of the conventions around meal-taking. However, some of the benefits of "delay" and not "grazing or pounce" may be lost to me.

THE TASTE FOR SWEETNESS IN OUR BUILT-IN TASTE-BUDS
MY BUILT-IN BIOLOGY

Our taste for sweetness is built into our taste buds. Salty-sweet-sour-bitter-savory are the five known taste bud tastes. Fat may be another taste. Natural scientists have asked why there are these tastes. What do they do for us human beings? Why did they come about? They believe that the savoury sense helped our ancestors to detect quality protein in foods. The sour sensation can be a sign that a food may have gone rotten; it could contain harmful bacteria. The bitter sense, another protective taste, was a good sign that plants that may contain poison. The protective taste buds would have helped our ancestors avoid eating potentially dangerous foods. The sweet taste buds, sensing sweetness in fruits and sweet leaves, would provide pleasant taste sensations, rewarding brains with pleasant taste, as well as bodies with quick energy from glucose.

Humans have gravitated toward sweetness thus eating fruits and sweet leaves. Eating fruits and sweet leaves provides quick energy from glucose. Then humans figured out how to store sweetness in foods so that the taste for sweetness might be satisfied when fresh fruit is not available. Dried fruit, dried vegetables, cured meats preserve food and are used in wintertime when fresh food is not available. The taste for sweetness has been met with these means until the coming of table sugar and artificial sweeteners.

Before 1650, there was no 'table sugar' in America, England or the rest of the world. Imagine. Table sugar came as ships sailed from Europe to the Caribbean Islands with the Trade Winds across the Atlantic, and picked up refined cane sugar, slaves, and rum. The ships sailed north to America on the Trade Winds and carried the cargo, bringing the sugar, slaves and rum to America. Then the ships sailed on the Trade Winds back across the Atlantic, bringing the cane sugar to the tables in England. There was a time before people put table sugar in their tea, before sugar bowls, and before the many confections made with refined table sugar. (*Sweetness & Power*, Sidney Mintz)

The market price of the commodity sugar has not declined in three centuries. The taste for "sweetness" has grown around the world. The taste buds for sweetness are built in to our evolutionary history. They insured that we would gravitate to foods that had sucrose for energy and survival. The taste buds for "sweetness" are built in.

The taste for sugar created new industries around the worlds. Refined sugar was at first the luxury of the aristocracy who showed wealth in their display of confections such as fancy cakes. Gradually increased manufacture made sugar available to the masses as a cheap source of calories.

The taste for "sweetness" created a new market for "sweeter" products. "Sweetness" was sold. New agricultural and chemical manufacturing methods created a means for producing "sweetness" under other names for sugar. These chemical forms of sweetness could be manufactured less expensively than refined sugar. They now compete with sugar cane on the world market as an ingredient additive because they are less expensive as an additive than cane sugar. (RuddCenter/Yale for Obesity & Food Addictions, http:// www.ruddcenteryale.org).

Meals without Sugar - One Accommodation to Live Well with All the Available Sweetness in My Culture

One accommodation to live well with all the available sweetness in my culture is to eat meals without sugar.

In 1953 Alcoholics Anonymous identified "the phenomenon of craving" in the book *Alcoholics Anonymous* (Alcoholics Anonymous, 1953). Called "an obsession of the mind and an allergy of the body" in talking about the craving for alcohol, the authors provided a clue to what many would identify as the "phenomenon of craving" around sweetness.

Whether it is the built-in deep system that prompts us human beings to have a taste for sweetness, brain-reward systems to sweetness, the constant exposure to food that makes me respond with "availability of food and opportunity to eat!" or the constant availability of sweetness in my culture, either glucose or other artificial sweetener foods, meals without sugar and with weighed and measured ingredients are one way of making an accommodation to too much available sweetness or too much available food.

What Do I Get from Standard Measures & Standard Measurements?

The rule of 'Standard Measures' was secured in England in *The Magna Carta* in the year 1212 as a right. The Barons, who owned property in England and managed crops grown by the serfs, obtained from King George an agreement – there would now be a standard measure used for goods sold and traded. People and merchants could trade throughout the land on a standard amount they would get for a certain price. Standard measures made trade increasingly possible, nationally and internationally (*The Magna Carta*, 1212).

Standard measures made the exchange of information increasingly possible. Standard measures made the duplication of scientific experiments possible. With standard measures, scientists could record, share and understand information across peoples, lands, and languages. Standard measures increasingly made science, medicine, and agriculture more precise. Where one erroneous measurement can distort an experiment's processes and results, and render the findings useless, standard measurements offer precision. Results can be duplicated.

In agriculture and in medicine standard measurements are vitally necessary.

With standard measures, we can compare prices based on measures. Standard measures allow us to duplicate cooking recipes or trade information about food portions and ingredients. Standard measures allow us to communicate about the portions of food we eat.

WEIGHING & MEASURING – ONE ACCOMMODATION TO LIVE WELL WITH ALL THE POWERS OF ADVERTISING - AVAILABILITY – EXPOSURE IN MY CULTURE

The powers of advertising – availability – exposure – around food – are great. Each of you can testify to these powers as they speak to you personally. Images flash on the television screen, parade in bright colors and shapes before you in grocery store aisles and shelves. They are powers of advertising – availability and exposure. They exert a power of imagination and scale on me. The images may take up my focus excluding other things I might focus on. They may loom large, as the only thing I focus on, or as all the available food in the world I must consume now and quickly. I may imagine and project imaginations onto these food items.

My powers of desire, great as a human being, may become focused on the entertainment value of these images or the substances, excluding higher level thinking or causing me to exercise my powers of desire to excess.

My powers of meditation and spirit can be used by me to foster to a sense of balance and sanity - "sanitus" - sound health body and mind – perspective and scale – reality – true need – true purpose.

THE SCIENCE & SPIRIT OF MEALS - ONE ACCOMMODATION TO LIVE WELL WITH MY DEEP SYSTEM OPERATING & IN MY HUMAN CULTURE

By planning and having meals vs. pounce or grazing,

* I reject instant gratification, and cultivate delayed gratification, by planning and preparing meals. I use my mind.

- I reject isolation from the food preparation process or the food industry's programmed disembodiment of eating from the human situation, and cultivate connection with my food.
- I reject the 24/7 opportunity to eat.
- I reject any fear that food and my opportunity to eat will never come again.
- I reject the idea that I must eat more than necessary because another opportunity will not come.
- I reject eating un-fresh food.
- I limit my grocery shopping experiences to specific times. I limit my exposure to food. .
- I am not in a rush. Because I have planned, I have the safety and security of knowing another meal is coming.
- I have the safety and security of knowing what will be in my meal.
- I foster a feeling – I am safe and secure. I know that another meal is coming and has been planned for.
- I eat meals. By eating my meals, I avoid excess hunger that would drive me to wildness.
- I practice clear thinking. I am part of community. I live not for myself alone. I am part of something greater than I am.
- I plan. I use my mind. I exercise my intelligence.
- I enjoy wholeness in appreciating the social rituals and meanings around meal preparation - planning the food shopping, choosing the freshest and best ingredients, taking the time to cook the meal, taking the time to eat and enjoy the meal, finishing the meal. Food and meal-taking is precious to me.
- I show how food and meal-taking is precious to me . I show it by having no phones, smart phones, or texting during meals; no television during meals; always having water in a glass on the table, cultivating safety and security; speaking respectfully in my mind's eye to myself and to others.

I find accommodations to live well and be well with my deep systems operating and in my human culture. I use what my ancestors used - meals - to help me. It helped them, delay immediate gratification, plan, and foster the social instinct. Where the bonds of the tribe in hunting, delay and group meals were originally formed, I too can use delay and my intelligence. I plan, I use my intelligence. "For God after all gave us our minds to use." (*Alcoholics Anonymous*, 1953.) This is *The 'Science and Spirit 'of Meals vs. Pounce or Grazing.*

This essay is called "The 'Science & Spirit' of Meals". It explains how hunger is a vital instinct with a purpose. Eating grows from my biology and meal-taking has grown from my social roots, as a cooperating thinking human being.

What about my spiritual roots and the spiritual experience of meal-taking? For many meal-taking involves, either explicitly said as a "Grace" or implicitly as a thought or silent prayer, acknowledging the Creator or the Great Reality.

William James in "The Varieties of Religious Experience" says that a spiritual or religious experience involves the belief that a higher power has our personal good at heart. He says in that series of lectures from his study of people, that his study is based on empirical or observed experience, that he observes the spiritual experience described by people.

When people say a Grace at meal-time, they ask that the food be used to their good. There is a hope in prayer for a personal contact for a personal good. We may "use" prayer in hope for that personal contact or good, or as affirmation of that personal good.

Meal-taking and the practices around food choices, food preparation, portions, sharing, pause, and behavior, whether eating alone or with others, is spiritual experience for me and for many - hoping that the meal may be used personally to my good, and that I may serve the Creator or the Great Reality.

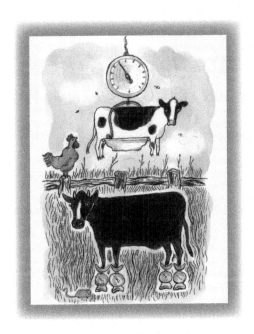

CHAPTER 6
Who's Cooking?
I'm Cooking

WHO'S COOKING? I'M COOKING

I Cook. I Weigh and Measure Using Cups and Scales. I Eat What I have Cooked and Measured. 'Peace of mind on a plate.' This cookbook is a cookbook. It is designed so 'I' can focus on cooking for my self-care, knowing the ingredients, and the amounts.' I aim to put some order in my life, for my preservation. I weigh and measure ingredients and portions. We cook. We share how we cook and eat. We prepare for, shop for, cook, and eat meals. Another meal is coming.

WHO CARES? I CARE FOR MY OWN FOOD ~ COOK ~ MEASURE

I Care. I Care for My Own Food – Cook – Measure. The contributors care for their own food. They care to benefit others who might learn and benefit from what they do.

Who's Eating? I'm Eating.
Sometimes Others are Eating With Me.

Everything Is Measured in Single Portions. I Double Recipes As Needed ~ When Cooking With Others.

I Measure Liquid Measures in Teaspoons-Tablespoons
& Cup Measurements'
Amounts Measured in Liquid/Fluid Ounces=Volume

Here, the standard fluid ounce measures apply, using cups and measuring spoons. The standard dry weight measures apply, using scales or digital scale. The Recipes & Sample Food Plans indicate whether the ingredient or portion is a liquid measure or a dry measure. The fluid ounce is defined as a unit of volume or capacity in the U.S. Customary System that equals 29.57 milliliters or 1.804 cubic inches. An ounce of weight is NOT a fluid ounce. Recipes measure ingredients either in liquid volume using teaspoon, tablespoon, and cups, or in dry weight using scales and ounces.

When the recipe gives a "Teaspoon, Tablespoon or Cup" measurement, it means you measure the ingredient using a Teaspoon, Tablespoon or a Measuring Cup.

A pinch/dash = less than 1/8 teaspoon
1 teaspoon = 1/3 tablespoon
1 1/2 teaspoon = 1/2 tablespoon
3 teaspoons = 1 tablespoon
1/4 cup = 4 tablespoons
1/3 cup = 5 tablespoons + 1 teaspoon
1/2 cup = 8 tablespoons
1 cup (dry ingredients) = 16 tablespoons
1 cup (liquid) = 8 ounces
1 1/2 cup = 12 ounces
2 cups (liquid) = 16 ounces or 1 pint or 1/2 quart
4 cups (liquid) = 1 quart
4 quarts (liquid) = 1 gallon

I MEASURE DRY MEASUREMENTS IN DRY WEIGHT SCALE OUNCE MEASUREMENTS

AMOUNTS MEASURED IN OUNCES = WEIGHT

AMOUNTS MEASURED IN DRY MEASURE = WEIGHT

When the recipe gives an "Ounce" measurement, it means you weigh the ingredient using a Digital Scale or Scale. If a Digital Scale is not available, you may measure the serving portion (.50 oz. or 4 ozs. or 8 ozs.) by using the equivalent measure with tablespoons or cups.

1/4 ounce = 1/2 tablespoon or .25 oz.

1/2 ounce = 1 tablespoon or .50 oz.

1 ounce = 2 tablespoons or 1.00 oz.

2 ounces = 4 tablespoons or 2.00 ozs.

4 ounces = 8 tablespoons or 4.00 ozs.

8 ounces = 1 cup or 16 tablespoons or 1/2 pound or 8.00 ozs.

12 ounces = 1 1/2 cup or 24 tablespoons or 3/4 pound or 12.00 ozs.

16 ounces = 2 cups or 32 tablespoons or 1 pound or 16.00 ozs.

32 ounces = 4 cups or 64 tablespoons or 2 pounds or 1 quart or 32.00 ozs.

64 ounces = 8 cups or 128 tablespoons or 2 pounds or 1 gallon or 64.00 ozs.

TO WEIGH AN INGREDIENT IN DIGITAL SCALE OUNCES

1. Place a piece of clean wax paper or clear wrap on the scale.
2. Press Clear or Zero out the Digital Scale so it begins on 0.00 oz.
3. Place your ingredient or food on the Digital Scale until the weighed amount is reached.

To Combine Weighed Ingredients Using a Digital Scale

1. Place a piece of clean wax paper or clear wrap or a bowl for weighing or combining ingredients on the scale.
2. Press Clear or Zero out the Digital Scale so it begins on 0.00 oz.
3. Place your ingredient or food on the Digital Scale until the weighed amount is reached. Leave the ingredients in the combining bowl on the digital scale.
4. Press Clear or Zero out the Digital Scale so it begins again on 0.00 oz.
5. Add the new ingredient until the new ingredient amount is reached.

For example: Salmon Salad

1. Put the combining bowl on the digital scale.
2. Zero out the digital scale so it now weighs 0.00 with the combining bowl on it.
3. Add 4 ozs. salmon until the digital scale shows 4.00 ozs.
4. Leave the combining bowl with the salmon on the digital scale
5. Zero out the digital scale so it now weighs 0.00 with the combining bowl on it.
6. Add 1 oz. chopped onion until the digital scale shows 1.00 oz.
7. Leave the combining bowl with the salmon and onion on the digital scale.
8. Zero out the digital scale so it now weighs 0.00 with the combining bowl on it.
9. Add 3 ozs. chopped green pepper until the digital scale shows 3 ozs.
10. Leave the combining bowl with the salmon and onion and chopped green pepper on the digital scale.
11. You now have 4 ozs. salmon, 1 oz chopped onion, 3 ozs. chopped green pepper.
12. Add 1 ½ tsp. mayonnaise, olive oil, or other oil.
13. Toss.

    Measured Portion : 4 ozs. protein ~. 4 ozs. raw vegetable ~ 1 1/2 serving oil.

To Convert from Fluid Ounces to Weighed Amounts if Necessary

If a digital scale is not available to weigh, or you want to convert from weight to volume – dry weight to liquid measurement or tablespoons or cups, you may use the simple equivalents given above - dry weight to liquid measurement or tablespoons or cups. Converting from fluid ounces to weight, or weight to fluid ounces, is vital to any science or agriculture experiment. It is usually carried out to two decimal places of weight for precise measurement. It is not necessary in most cases when measuring food ingredients or portions. However, converting from fluid ounces to weight, or weight to fluid ounces, can be done to two decimal places for cooking by consulting: http://www.onlineconversion.com/weight_volume_cooking.htm

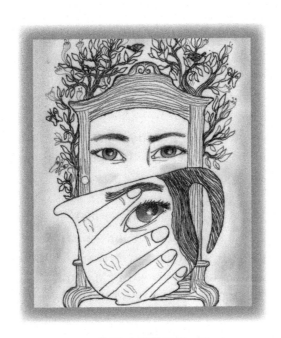

CHAPTER 7
What's In It — What Isn't In It
Ingredients - Foods

NO SUGAR-WHEAT-FLOUR

No Sugar or Other Forms of Sugar
No Concentrated Fruit Juices
No Wheat
No Flour
No Whole Grain Flour
No Soy Flour or Texturized Vegetable Protein
No Food Starch or Modified Food Starch
No Extracts with Alcohol
No Alcohol or Sugar Alcohols for Cooking or Drinking
Fat-Oil is Measured
Non-Aerosol Oil Mist Used

How To Read Label 'Ingredients'?

Fructose, High Fructose Corn Syrup (HFCS), Corn Syrup, Dextrin Maltitol, Maltodextrin, or another form of sucrose or starch filler additive may have been added to the food – even if the label says "sugar free" or "natural". In addition to the naturally occurring carbohydrates listed on the "nutrition" part of the label, there may be other forms of sugar and starch filler additives added, listed in the "ingredients" portion of the label.

'Natural' is a "new" term to make the consumer feel the ingredients are "good for you" or come from a grown food. However, the term 'natural' on the packaging or 'ingredient' label <u>does not mean</u> there is no form of sugar added. Fructose, High fructose corn syrup (HFCS), Corn Syrup, Dextrin, Maltitol, Maltodextrin, or another form of sucrose or starch filler additive may be added to the food (www.wikipedia.com).

There are naturally occurring carbohydrates in a food. Do not confuse these with added sucrose, fructose, high fructose corn syrup (HFCS), corn syrup, dextrin, malitol, maltodextrin or another form of sucrose or starce filler that may have been added to a food and will be listed on the ingredients portion of the label.

How To Read Label 'Nutrition'
What Do 'Carbohydrate Grams' or 'Sugar Grams" Mean?

'Nutrition' on the label indicates the grams of protein, fat (saturated fats and unsaturated fats), and carbohydrates (naturally occurring sugar and added forms of sugar if they are included on the 'ingredients' part of the label.) Where there are no other forms of sugar added on the 'ingredients' part of the label, there are still carbohydrates (naturally occurring sugars or carbohydrates) in the food. We all need naturally occurring carbohydrates in food (www.wikipedia.com).

There are naturally occurring carbohydrates in a food. Do not confuse these with sucrose, fructose, high fructose corn syrup (HFCS), corn syrup, dextrin, malitol, maltodextrin or another form of sucrose or starce filler that may have been added to a food and will be listed on the ingredients portion of the label.

Ingredient & Serving Amounts in the Recipes

What Are the Foods?

What is a Serving Amount?

All recipes give a single serving amount of the ingredient. The recipes will help you with weighing and measuring ingredient amounts and single serving amounts for meals. The number of servings for a food group for a meal for a specific plan of eating is listed on the specific Sample Plans of Eating.

» FRUITS

The recipes include these fruits. The recipes use these quantities as a single serving portion – 6 ozs. or as otherwise specified.

Apple – 6 ozs. or 1 med.

Apricots – 6 ozs. or 3 med.

Banana – ½ small (infrequently) or 3 ozs.

Blackberries - ½ cup

Blueberries - ½ cup

Boysenberries - 1 cup

Cantaloupe - ½ whole or 6 ozs.

Canned Fruit – ½ cup (example - Pineapple, unadvised or in unsweetned juice only)

Casaba Melon - ¼ whole or 6 ozs.

Cherries – 10 cherries (not often) or 3 ozs.

Clementine - 6 ozs.

Cranberries – 6 ozs.

Gooseberries – 6 ozs.

Grapefruit - ½ whole or 6 ozs.

Grapes – 10 grapes (infrequently) or 3 ozs.

Honeydew Melon - ¼ whole or 6 ozs.

Kiwi – 6 ozs. or 3 smLemons – 2 whole

Limes – 2 whole

Mango – 6 ozs.

No Fruit Juices

Orange - 1 whole or 6 ozs.

Papaya – 6 ozs.

Peach – 6 ozs.

Pear – 6 ozs.

Pineapple - 6 ozs. (fresh, infrequently) ½ cup or 4 ozs. canned (no juice)

Plum – 6 ozs.

Raspberries - ½ cup

Rhubarb – 6 ozs.

Strawberries – 6 ozs.

Tangerine – 6 ozs.

Watermelon – 6 ozs. (infrequently)

» DAIRY & DAIRY SUBSTITUTES

The recipes include dairy and dairy-free substitutes. Dairy and dairy substitutes may be used as a dairy serving or as a protein serving. Dairy and dairy substitutes include milk and yogurt with less than 2% fat, hard cheese, and soft cheese, 1/3 cup nonfat dry milk = 5 tbs. = 1 cup liquid; unsweetened soymilk, 2 tbs. soy protein (no Texturized Vegetable Protein, contains flour); 4 ozs. tofu, tempeh; 4 egg whites; 1 cup buttermilk

Milk (less than 2% fat content)

Yogurt (less than 2% fat content; no sugar, plain)

Dry Powdered Milk – 1/3 cup dry = 5 tbs – 1 cup liquid

» PROTEINS - ANIMAL & SOY PROTEINS

These recipes include these animal and soy proteins.

Beef 4 oz.

Chicken 4 oz.

Dairy as Protein (may be used as a protein)

Milk or Milk Substitute (unsweetened soy milk; soy protein)

Skim, or less than 2% - 1 cup

Hard cheese – 2 ozs.

Soft cheese – cottage cheese, ricotta, farmer's cheese – 4 ozs.

Dairy Substitutes (2 ozs. soy powder, 4 ozs. tofu, tempeh, 4 egg whites)

Dried beans (when used as a protein vs. starch) 1 cup, cooked

Eggs 2 med. (4 egg whites)

Fish 4 oz.

Hot dogs (not sugar cured) 4 oz.

Lamb 4 oz.

Pork 4 oz.

Shellfish 4 oz.

Tofu or Tembeh – Vegetable Protein

Turkey 4 oz.

Veal 4 oz.

Vegetarian protein (Tofu, Tempeh) - 4 ozs.

No Texturized Vegetable Protein - contains flour

Men & Pregnant Women especially should check with your healthcare practitioner for your serving needs.

» PROTEIN SERVING SIZE

Beef - 4 ozs.

Bacon – 2 ozs.

Buttermilk - 1 cup

Cheese - 2 oz. (hard cheese)

Cheese – ½ cup or 4 ozs. (soft cheese, cottage, ricotta, farmers)

Chicken - 4 ozs.

Clams - 4 ozs.

Crab - ½ cup.

Cold Cuts - 2 slices.

Cottage Cheese - ½ cup.

Eggs – 2 large

Fish - 4 ozs.

Frankfurters – 2 links – 4 ozs.

Ham - 4 ozs.

Heart - 4 ozs.

Kidney - 4 ozs.

Lamb - 4 ozs.

Liver - 4 ozs.

Lobster - 4 ozs.

Milk – skim or less than 2% - 1 cup - 8 fl. ounces

Nuts – 2 ozs.

Oysters - 4 ozs.

Pork - 4 ozs.

Salmon - ½ cup or 4 ozs.

Sardines - ½ cup

Shrimp - 4 ozs.

Soyburger - 4 ozs.

Soynut Butter – 2 ozs.

Soy Nuts - 2 ozs.

Sausage – 4 ozs.

Soybeans – 1 cup

Soy Protein - 2 ozs.

Steak - 4 ozs.

Tempeh – 4 ozs.

Tofu – 4 ozs.

Tongue - 4 ozs.

Tuna - ½ cup

Turkey - 4 ozs.

Veal - 4 ozs.

Yogurt, low fat plain - 1 cup

» STARCHES/GRAINS

Starches/Grains consist of the grain family, certain vegetables that are counted as starches, and starchy vegetables that may be counted either as a starch or as a starchy vegetable.

» GRAINS -

Serving amounts for Starches/Grains are based on plan of eating. See Plans of Eating 1-6. In Plan of Eating 7, Starches/Grains are not used.

1 ozs. (dry weight) = ½ cup or 4 ozs. (liquid-cooked)

2 ozs. (dry weight) = 1 cup or 8 ozs. (liquid cooked) Servings based on plan of eating.

Amaranth
Brown Rice
Buckwheat Groats – Kasha
Cream of Rye
Grits
Millet
Oat Bran
Whole Grain Oats
Cooked Oatmeal
Dry Raw Oatmeal
Steel Cut Oats
Quinoa

» STARCHES/
» VEGETABLE STARCHES

These Vegetables are Starches –
½ cup (liquid-cooked) or 4 ozs. (weighed) They are counted as starches in servings. In Plan of Eating 7, these vegetables are not allowed.

Corn – 4 ozs. or ½ cup or 1 ear
Peas – 4 ozs. or ½ cup
Potato – 4 ozs. or ½ cup
Sweet Potato/Yam – 4 ozs. or ½ cup

» BEANS & LEGUMES

Beans and legumes have more carbohydrates per ounce than animal or dairy protein. Bean and legume recipes are included in the Starches/Grains Recipes. Vegans and vegetarians especially need to consult with your health practitioner on servings.

Serving amounts for Beans/Legumes as Starches/Grains are based on plan of eating. See Plans of Eating 1-6. In Plan of Eating 7, Beans/Legumes & Starches/Grains are not used.

Beans: lima, navy, all dried beans -
1 starch/grain = ½ cup or 4 ozs. (liquid - cooked) or
2 starch/grains = 1 cup or 8 ozs. (liquid – cooked)

Aduki Beans
Black Beans
Black-Eyed Peas
Cannelini Beans
Chick Peas/Garbanzo Beans
Kidney Beans
Lentils
Lima Beans
Mung Beans
Navy Beans
Pinto Beans
Red Beans
Soy Beans
Split Peas

» STARCHY VEGETABLES -

» These vegetables may be counted as a starchy vegetable - ½ cup (liquid-cooked) or 4 ozs. (weighed) or as a starch

Baked potato (white) - 1 sm., 4 oz.

Beets – 4 ozs. or ½ cup

Carrots – 4 ozs. or ½ cup

Corn (ear) - 1 med.

Corn (kernel) - 4 ozs. or ½ cup

Mashed potatoes (white) (nothing added) - 4 ozs. or ½ cup

Mashed yams (nothing added) - 4 ozs. or ½ cup

Onions – 4 ozs. or ½ cup

Parsnips - 4 ozs. or ½ cup

Peas, dried - 4 ozs. or ½ cup

Peas, green - 4 ozs. or ½ cup

Pumpkin – 4 ozs. or ½ cup

Rutabagas – 4 ozs. or ½ cup

Sweet potato - 1 sm., 4 ozs. or ½ cup

Water Chestnuts – 4 ozs. or ½ cup.

Wheat Germ - 1/8 cup = 2 tbs.

Winter Squash – 4 ozs.

  Acorn Squash – 4 ozs.

  Butternut Squash – 4 ozs.

  Hubbard Squash – 4 ozs.

  Spaghetti Squash – 4 ozs.

  Turban Squash – 4 ozs.

Yam - 4 ozs. or ½ cup

» VEGETABLES - RAW & COOKED

Different Plans of Eating call for different serving amounts. Serving amounts range from 1 cup or 8 ozs. to 1 ½ cup or 12 ozs. to 2 cups or 16 ozs.

Artichoke

Arugula

Asparagus

Bean Sprouts

Green Beans

Yellow Wax Beans

Bamboo Shoots

Beet Greens

Bok Choy

Broccoli

Broccoli Rabe

Brussels Sprouts

Cabbage

Chinese Cabbage

Collard Greens

Cauliflower

Celery

Cucumber

Dill Pickles (no sugar)

Eggplant

Endive

Escarole

Greens – Beet, Collard, Dandelion, Kale, Mustard

Jicama

Lettuce (no wheat grass)

Mushrooms

Okra

Onions

Parsley

Parsnips

Peppers – Red, Green, Yellow

Pimentos – Roasted Peppers

Radishes
Roasted Peppers
Sauerkraut
Snow Pea Pods
Spinach
Sprouts
Summer Squash
Tomatoes
Tomato Juice – Vegetable Juice (no sugar)
Yellow Squash, Summer
Watercress
Zucchini, Green Squash, Summer

» FATS - DRESSING - OILS

The 7 Sample Plans of Eating illustrated here show different daily fat allotments. We suggest you discuss and decide with your health practitioner and your sponsor what your daily fat allotment requirement is. Men & Pregnant Women especially should check with your healthcare practitioner on determining your needs.

Oil
Butter - Margarine
Mayonnaise

1 tsp. = 5 grams fat
2 tsp. = 10 grams fat
3 tsp. = 14-16 grams fat = 1 Tablespoon
10-15 Non-Aerosol Oil Mists = 1 tsp.
We found using Non-Aerosol Oil Mist that an oil mister will dispense 1 tsp. oil in 10-15 mists. See Chapter 11: Resources & Links for more information on measure values with Non-Aerosol Oil Mist and Press & Measure Oil Pumps and where they may be purchased.

» SEASONINGS ~ SPICES

These recipes use sugar-free, alcohol-free, flour free, starch free, wheat-free, spices and seasonings including, but not limited to allspice, non-sugar almond flavor, fresh basil, cayenne pepper, celery powder, chai spices, chili powder, cilantro, cinnamon stick, ground cinnamon, dill seed, dill weed, fresh garlic, garlic powder, garlic salt, lemon juice, lemon pepper, lime juice, mint, mustard, fresh nutmeg, ground nutmeg, onion powder, paprika, parsley, pepper, peppermint, rosemary, sage, salsa, sea salt, thyme, non-fat yogurt, fresh vanilla, non-alcohol vanilla.

See Chapter 8: Recipes for Spice Blend Recipes:
See Chapter 11: Resources & Links for information on no alcohol no sugar flavorings.

Barbecue Blend
Cajun Blend
Caribbean Blend
Country Blend
Fish & Seafood Herbs
French Blend
Herbes de Provence
Holiday Meat & Poultry Blend
Italian Blend
Mediterranean Blend
Middle Eastern Blend
Old Bay Seasoning
Pacific Rim Asian Blend
Sonoran Southwest Blend
Swedish Spice Blend
Texas Blend

2 egg whites = 1 egg

4 egg whites = 2 eggs

1/2 cup egg whites = 2 eggs

4 ozs. tofu = 1 dairy or protein

1 cup unsweetened soymilk = 1 dairy or protein

1 ozs. hard cheese = ½ dairy or protein

2 ozs. hard cheese = 1 dairy or protein

4 ozs. or ½ cup soft cheese = 1 dairy or protein

8 ozs. dairy = 1 protein

2 ozs. dry grain = 1 cup cooked grain

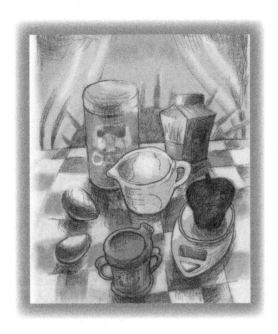

CHAPTER 8
Recipes

Fruits
Fruit with Dairy/Protein
Fruit with Dairy/Protein with Starch/Grain
Dairy /Protein & Dairy-Free Choices
Protein ~ Animal & Soy Protein
Starches/Grains & Beans/Legumes
Starchy Vegetables
Cooked Vegetables
Cooked Vegetables with Protein
Cooked Vegetables with Protein with Starch/Grain
Raw Vegetables
Raw Vegetables with Protein
Fats - Dressing - Oils - Sauces
Seasonings — Spice Blends - Condiments

Fruit

Apple - Baked Apple Glory

1. Remove core from apple.
2. Place apple in dish and sprinkle with cinnamon.
3. Add nutmeg and cinnamon to taste.
4. Bake in an a) oven roaster for about 20 minutes at 325 degrees, b) an oven for about 45 minutes at 350 degrees, c) in the microwave on high about 3 minutes.

- *1 large apple* • *1/2 tsp cinnamon*
- *1/2 tsp nutmeg*

Serving amount: 6 ozs. fruit

Apricots - Poached

1. Halve the fresh apricots.
2. Bring water to a boil.
3. Add vanilla flavor and poach till the apricots are just tender.
4. Poach either in water on stovetop or in microwave on high for 1 minute.
5. Serve cold.

- *3 medium apricots* • *2 cups water*
- *1/2 teaspoon vanilla extract*

Serving amount: 6 ozs. fruit

Blueberry Sauce

1. Mix ingredients.
2. Leave blueberries whole or smoosh-crush berries.
3. Cook in small pot on stovetop or heat in microwave 1 minute.

- *1/2 cup blueberries* • *2 tablespoons cold water*

Serving amount: 1/2 cup blueberries

Cantaloupe with Salt & Lemon

1. Prepare 6 ozs fresh cantelope by slicing, quartering and cutting into chunks or slices.
2. Sprinkle with lemon juice.
3. Dust with salt.

- *6 ozs. cantaloupe* • *1 tsp. fresh squeezed lemon*
- *1 dash salt from a salt shaker*

Serving amount: 6 ozs. fruit

Fruit

Citrus Fruit Salad

1. Peel and section grapefruit and oranges.
2. Mix and measure 6 ounces for one fruit serving.

___

• *1 grapefruit* • *2 oranges*

Serving amount: 6 ozs. fruit

Cranberry Relish Sauce

1. Put cranberries and orange in food processor.
2. Pulse food processor or blender lightly until fruit is minced into small pieces. Make sure it does not become liquid.
3. Add sweetener (optional).
4. Heat in a saucepan or microwave for 1-2 minutes.
5. Make sure sauce does not burn.
6. Add water if you want a more liquid sauce.
7. Add nutmeg, cinnamon or orange peel if you like.
8. Use 6 ozs. fruit per serving.

___

• *1 bag cranberries ~ sweetener (optional) ~ 1 navel orange*

Serving amount: 6 ozs. fruit

Cranberry Sauce

1. Rinse cranberries.
2. Peel, core, slice and finally chop apple.
3. Put the cranberries and apple in a saucepan, microwavable dish, or slow cooker, with the water.
4. Add sweetener (optional).
5. Cook the cranberries until they have popped and are hot and mushy. Be careful not to burn. Saucepan - estimated time - 5 minutes. Microwave - on High - estimated cooking time - 4 minutes. Slow cooker - on High - estimated cooking time 20 minutes. The longer you cook the thicker the sauce will become. You may add cinnamon, cloves, nutmeg or orange peel.
6. Use 6 ozs. of the cranberry sauce for a single portion. Freeze the rest.

___

• *1 bag cranberries ~ sweetener (optional) ~ 1 apple*

Serving amount: 6 ozs. fruit

Grapes, Frozen - Frozen Peach Slices - Frozen Apricot Slices

1. Select 10 grapes or weigh 6 ozs. peach.
2. Put in a freezer bag.
3. Freeze overnight.

___

• *10 red or green grapes or 6 ozs. peach or apricot*

Serving amount: 6 ozs. fruit

Fruit

Hot Spiced Tea

1. Put the tea bags, spices, and orange peel in a ceramic or glass container and pour the boiling water over them; cover and allow to steep for 5 minutes. 2. Strain the mixture. 3. Stir in the orange and lemon juices; reheat if necessary. You can also chill it and serve over ice for a refreshing iced tea.

• 2 tea bags • 14 whole cloves • 1 cinnamon stick
• 1 strip (about 3 inches) fresh orange zest
• 2 cups boiling water • 3/4 cup orange juice
• 1 1/2 tbs. lemon juice

Serving amount: 6 ozs. fruit

Iced Ginger-Orange Green Tea

1. In medium saucepan,
bring the water to boil.
2. In a ceramic container, pour the boiling water over the ginger and orange peel.
3. Add tea bags; cover,
and steep for 5 minutes.
4. Remove the tea bags,
ginger, and orange peel.
5. Add the orange juice
to the tea blend, and stir.
6. Put ice cubes in glasses, pour orange juice-tea blend over the ice, and serve. Makes 4 portions. Each portion equals 6 ozs. fruit

---

• 2 cups water • 1 tb. coarsely chopped ginger root or 1 tbs. ground ginger • 2 (1-inch) pieces orange zest • 4 green tea bags • 12 ozs. orange juice, chilled

Serving amount: 6 ozs. fruit

Orange or Grapefruit - Broiled

1. Take orange, cut in half and section like a grapefruit.
2. Broil for 2 minutes under broiler or heat in microwave for 2 minutes

---

• 1 medium orange • 1/2 tsp cinnamon, 1/2 tsp cloves (optional)

Serving amount: 6 ozs. fruit

Peachy Gingered Tea Homemade

1. Peel and core peach, cut in slices or cubes. Measure 6 ounces of pear.
2. Combine water, ginger, sweetener(optional and cinnamon in saucepan.
3. Bring to a boil, add the peach, reduce heat and simmer for 3 minutes. Strain ginger piec out of tea.
4. Serve warm or cold.

• 6 ozs. peach • 1 tbs. sliced fresh ginger or 1 tbs. ground ginger • 1 quart water • sweetener (optiona • 1/8 tsp. cinnamon or nutmeg

Serving amount: 6 ozs. fruit

Fruit

Orange - Sliced

1. Peel the orange or slice off the skin with a sharp knife so that the inner film of white is entirely removed.
2. Slice quite thinly.
3. Sprinkle with dash of cinnamon.
4. Heat or serve cold.
5. To heat, a) bake in oven roaster for 10 minutes at 325 degrees or b) microwave on high for 1 1/3 minutes.

• *1 medium orange* • *1/2 tsp cinnamon, 1/2 tsp cloves (optional)*

Poached Pear

1. Peel and core pear, cut in half. Measure 6 ounces of pear.
2. Combine water, sweetener and cinnamon in saucepan.
3. Bring to a boil, add the pear, reduce heat and simmer for 3 minutes.
4. Serve warm.

• *6 ozs. pear* • *1/2 cup water* • *sweetener (optional)* • *1/8 tsp. cinnamon or nutmeg*

Serving amount: 6 ozs. fruit

Rhubarb & Strawberries - Stewed - Warm or Chilled

1. Peel and cut rhubarb in 3 inch or 4-inch stalks. Discard the leaves.
2. Wash & take the tops off of fresh strawberries. You may use frozen rhubarb, with no sugar.
3. Put rhubarb and strawberries in a saucepan; add 2 cups water, and pinch salt (optional). Stew on stovetop until cooked and soft. Measure 6 ozs. fruit for 1 serving fruit. You may also arrange rhubarb and strawberries in 1 1/2-quart casserole dish with a cover. Add water and bake at 350 degrees until the rhubarb and strawberries are soft. Enjoy the aroma. May be measured and frozen in small containers and reheated as required.

• *1 1/2 pounds rhubarb* • *2 cups water*
• *2 cups strawberries* • *dash of salt. Measure 6 ozs serving.*

Serving amount: 6 ozs. fruit

Fruit with Dairy/Protein

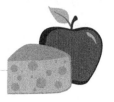

Apple Baked with Yogurt or Cottage Cheese

1. Peel, core and cut apple in small pieces.
2. Place cottage cheese on top of apple, top with cinnamon and sweetener. Bake at 350 degrees for 20 or Microwave for 1-2 minutes.

• *6 ozs. apple chopped* • *1/2 tsp. cinnamon*
• *1/2 cup cottage cheese*

Serving amount 6 ozs. fruit, 1 protein or dairy

Apple - Hot with Ricotta Cheese

1. Heat the apple in an oven, a microwave, or sautée it in a small pan.
2. Top with ricotta cheese and vanilla flavoring, cinnamon. The contrast between the hot apple and the cold ricotta is quite nice.

• *1 apple* • *2 ozs. ricotta cheese*

Serving amount: 6 ozs. fruit, 1 protein

Apple Nut Breakfast

1. Blend cheese until smooth.
2. Peel, core, and weigh apple.
3. Spoon cheese blend over apple and top with split soynuts.

• *3/8 c ricotta cheese* • *1 oz. split roasted soynuts*
• *6 ozs. apple pieces*

Serving amount: 6 ozs. fruit, 4 ozs. dairy or protein

Apple Omelet

1. Whip together eggs, water and first two spices.
2. Spray the fry pan with non-aerosol oil mist Heat pan.
3. Pour egg/spice mixture into pan. Cook a you would any omelet.
4. When the egg mixture is 1/2 or 3/4 done, add apple and cover again. Cook unti the apple has just about evaporated and caramelized.
5. Uncover the pan for a minute or two. Tur onto a plate. Garnish plate and omelet with cinnamon.

• *2 eggs (warmed up to room temperature)*
• *1 tbs water* • *1/4 tsp allspice* • *1/4 tsp nutmeg*
• *1/4 tsp cinnamon (for garnish)*
• *6 ozs. chopped fresh apple*

Serving amount: 6 ozs. fruit, 1 protein

Fruit with Dairy/Protein

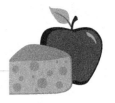

Apple - Un-Caramel Look-Alike Taste with Soynuts

1. Cut up your apple. Lay it on a dish.
2. Pour the 1 oz. gjetost cheese on top of the apple.
3. Add 1 oz. soy nut on top of it (either ground in a coffee grinder or whole).

- *1 apple* • *1 oz. ghetost cheese* • *1 oz. soy nuts*
- *cinnamon* • *1-2 tsp. no alcohol vanilla extract*

Serving amount : 6 ozs. fruit, 1 protein or dairy

Apple Slices with Soynut Butter

1. Weigh and measure apple.
2. Measure soynut butter. You may use I.M. Healthy Unsweetened Soynut Butter.
3. Spread apple slices with soynut butter.

- *6 ozs. fruit* • *4 ozs. soynut butter*

Serving amount: 6 ozs. fruit, 1 protein

Apple Smoothie

1. Put milk, apple and spices into a blender and blend to mix.

- *8 ozs. milk* • *6 ozs. frozen or fresh apple slices 1/4 tsp. cinnamon, 1/4 tsp. nutmeg, 1/4 tsp. cloves, 1.4 tsp. allspice*

Serving amount: 6 ozs. fruit, 1 protein

Blackberry or Blueberry Topping on Egg

1. Beat egg.
2. Pour into heated saute pan. (like making an omelet) on med-low heat. Allow egg to cook until no longer soupy, then flip the entire egg patty and cook other side. In separate bowl, mix cheese & fruit together. Spoon cheese mixture on top of egg patty.

- *1 egg*
- *1/4 cup (1 oz.) ricotta or cottage cheese*
- *6 ozs chopped apple or 1/2 cup blueberries or raspberries or blackberries*

Blueberries and Soynut Butter

1. Weigh and measure blueberries.
2. Warm in the microwave until hot and super juicy.
3. Then add 2 oz soynut butter.

- *6 ozs. frozen blueberries* • *2 ozs. soynut butter*

Serving amount: 6 ozs. fruit, 1 protein

Fruit with Dairy/Protein

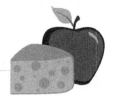

Blueberry, Strawberry or Pineapple Ricotta Frozen Cheesecake

1. Start with a serving of 1/2 cup blueberries - or 1 cup strawberries or 1/2 cup crushed pineapple. The fruit can either be fresh, frozen and thawed, or canned - as long as it is the abstinent kind of course, no sugar added.
2. Add 1/2 cup ricotta cheese.
3. Combine all ingredients so far in a small, freezer-proof container. It is not necessary to blend or mix completely. Mixing well with a fork should be sufficient.
4. Put the container in the freezer. It usually takes about two hours in the freezer to reach the right consistency, but you can experiment. Don't worry if you over freeze - 20-40 seconds in the microwave should fix it. The microwave method also works if you want to make several in advance and leave them in the freezer.

• *1/2 cup blueberries or 1 cup strawberries or 1/2 cup pineapple* • *1/2 cup ricotta Cheese*

Serving amount: 6 ozs. fruit, 1 protein or dairy

Egg-Sausage Rutti Tutti Sweet Surprise

1. Cube sausage patties and cook in saute pan until slightly browned.
2. Beat egg and pour into heated saute pan (like making an omelet) on medium-low heat. Allow egg to cook until no longer soupy, then flip the entire egg patty and cook other side.
3. Once cooked, place egg patty on plate and top with sausage and cooked fruit.

• *1 egg* • *2 oz. breakfast sausage patties (cubed)*
• *1 serving of fruit*

Serving amount: 6 ozs. fruit, 1 protein

Fruit Nice Cream

1. Put all ingredients in a blender, and blend until mixed thoroughly.
2. Turn on your yogurt maker, so the frozen bowl is spinning.
3. Pour the mixture into the top hole of the frozen yogurt maker.
4. Let the yogurt maker spin until the blade no longer moves the mixture. This can be served immediately or stored frozen. A summer favorite!

• *1/4 cup cottage cheese or 1/2 cup plain yogurt*
• *1 cup milk* • *1 cup frozen strawberries*
• *peaches, or 1 chilled peeled apple, or 1/2 cup frozen blueberries*

Serving amount: 6 ozs. fruit, 1 protein, 1 cup dairy

Fruit with Dairy/Protein

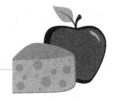

Gjetost Cheese and Apple Baked

1. Cut apple in chunks.
2. Cut cheese in small slices or chunks and place on top of apple.
3. Top with cinnamon and sweetener or coffee syrup.
4. Microwave for 30 seconds or until cheese is melted.

• *2 ozs. Gjetost cheese* • *1 apple* • *cinnamon*

Serving amount: 6 ozs. fruit, 1 protein or dairy

Lemon Mousse

1. Mix lemon juice, grated lemon peel and flavorings and sweetener.
2. Put all the ingredients into a food processor; process until smooth.
3. Refrigerate in a covered container for at least 1 hour before serving. Makes 4 portions. Each portion equals 1 protein.

• *1 1/2 cups mashed silken firm tofu (12 ozs.)*
• *sweetener (optional)*
• *2 tbs. unsweetened soynot butter*
• *1 tbs. lemon zest* • *1 tsp. pure vanilla extract*
• *1 tsp. pure lemon extract* • *garnish (optional lemon slices)*

Serving amount: 6 ozs. fruit, 1 protein or dairy

Lemon Sherbet Ice Cube Tray Method

1. Mix lemon juice, grated lemon peel and flavorings and sweetener.
2. Add to cold milk.
3. Mix well.
4. Pour into ice cube trays.
5. Freeze for 1 1/2 hours or until sloshy. Take out and stir in the ice cube tray at this point to break up ice crystals.
6. Put back in freezer and freeze for another 1 1/2 hour. Delicious. Makes 2 portions. Each portion equals 1 dairy, 3 ozs. or 1/2 fruit

---

• *2 cups milk* • *2/3 cup lemon juice or juice of two fresh lemons* • *1 tbs. grated fresh lemon peel rind* • *1 tsp. lemon extract of flavoring* • *sweetener (optional).*

Serving amount: 3 ozs. or 1/2 fruit, 1 cup dairy

Orange Dreamsicle - Frozen

1. Blend all ingredients in food processor.
2. Freeze overnight

• *1 cup plain lowfat yogurt*
• *1 medium peeled and quartered orange*
• *vanilla flavoring (no alcohol)*

Serving amount: 6 ozs. fruit, 1 protein or dairy

Fruit with Dairy/Protein

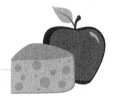

Orange Broiled With Strained Yogurt

1. Measure 1 cup yogurt before straining.
2. Strain 1 cup of yogurt overnight in a strainer lined with a coffee filter.
3 Place 1/2 cup (4 ozs.) fresh pineapple or 6 ozs fresh orange under broiler.
4. Place yogurt mixture on top of orange and serve. May be prepared with pineapple instead of orange.

• *6 ozs fresh orange sliced* • *1 cup yogurt. May be prepared with 1/2 cup or 4 ozs fresh or canned with no-sugar pineapple.*

Serving amount: 6 ozs. fruit, 1 dairy or protein

Orange Ricotta Pudding

1. Peel and cut oranges into bite size pieces.
2. Add ricotta, vanilla flavor (no-alcohol).
3. Strawberries, blueberries, or apple sprinkled with cinnamon can be substituted.

• *1 navel orange (no seeds)* • *4 ozs. or 1/2 cup ricotta cheese*

Serving amount: 6 ozs. fruit, 1 protein or dairy

Peach - Nectarine Shake Smoothie

1. Place all ingredients into blender, blend until smooth. You can use 6oz. frozen peaches.

• *6 ozs. sliced peaches* • *1/2 cup frozen skim milk*
• *1/2 cup skim milk*

Serving amount: 6 ozs. fruit, 1 cup dairy

Peaches and Cream

1. Mix ricotta cheese and frozen peaches in a blender, or food processor, and chop until fine, but not blended smooth.
2. Stir in extract.
3. Top with soy nuts.

• *2 ozs. ricotta cheese* • *1 oz. roasted split soy nuts* • *1 cup frozen peaches with no syrup added*
• *1 tbs. vanilla flavoring (no alcohol)*

Serving amount: 6 ozs. fruit, 1 protein or dairy, 1/4 protein or dairy

Fruit with Dairy/Protein

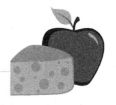

Pineapple Cottage Cheese Mix

1. Mix together and cook in microwave until warm or eat cold if that is your preference.

• *4 ozs. diced pineapple* • *1/2 cup cottage cheese*

Serving amount: 6 ozs. fruit, 4 ozs. protein

Pineapple Ricotta No Sugar Sorbet

1. The night before you are ready to use, take your pineapple, your ricotta, blend in the blender.
2. After blended, put up in a bowl or glass and freeze overnight.
3. Ready to use in the morning.

• *1/2 cup pineapple* • *4 ozs, ricotta*

Serving amount: 6 ozs. fruit, 1 protein or dairy

Root Beer Moat Sherbet Float

1. Peel the apple, and chop it up into 1/2 inch cubes. Put in a blender. Blend.
2. Turn on frozen yogurt maker. Pour ingredients slowly into top hole of yogurt maker. Stop the yogurt maker when mixture thickens.
4. Serve immediately, or freeze for serving later. Pour desired amount of diet root beer in the serving dish. Other extract flavors and seltzer with no alcohol, no sugar work, too!

• *1 cup milk* • *1/4 cup cottage cheese or 1/2 cup plain yogurt* • *6 ozs.chilled apple* • *1 can or bottle of chilled diet root beer or 1 cup seltzer with no alcohol, no sugar, lemon, maple or other extract* • *1 tsp. vanilla extract*

Serving amount: 6 ozs. fruit, 1/2 or 2 ozs. protein, 1 cup dairy

Fruit with Dairy/Protein

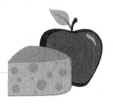

Soymilk Fruit Shake

1. Mix with a blender. I use frozen fruit in no-sugar or juices. Also frozen fruit is great because the shake comes out thick and frothy. 2. Pour into a pleasing glass and enjoy.

• *4 ozs. yogurt* • *8 ozs. unsweetened soymilk*
• *6 ozs. frozen blueberries* • *6 vanilla flavoring*

Serving amount: 6 ozs. fruit, 1 cup dairy, 1/2 or 2 ozs. protein

Strawberry - Apple - Orange Julius Smoothie

1. Mix ingredients in a blender. Makes a smoothie.
2. Good for different combinations of dairy and fruit blended in the blender.
3. Possible combinations: orange, strawberries alone.

• *6 ozs. frozen berries* • *1 cup skim milk or 1 cup unsweetened soymilk. Makes 1 portion. Equals: 6 ozs. fruit, 1 cup dairy*

Serving amount : 6 ozs. fruit, 1 cup diary or dairy-free substitute

Strawberry Cheese Squares

1. Add the extract to yogurt and stir.
2. Chop fruit finely in food processor.
3. Grind soy nuts into powder.
4. In 5 x 5 dish, fold fruit into yogurt, leaving pockets.
5. Sprinkle ground soy nuts on top, and freeze until firm.
6. Let thaw until semi-frozen before serving.

• *7/8 cup yogurt* • *1/2 oz. roasted salted soy nuts* • *1 cup frozen strawberries* • *1 1/2 tbs. no alcohol vanilla flavoring*

Serving amount: 6 ozs. fruit, 1 protein

Strawberry Pineapple Tropical Delight

1. Measure and combine all fruit and protein in food processor.
2. Blend until mixed well. Pour into shallow plastic dish with cover.
3. Place in freezer for at least 4 hours.
4. Top with coffee syrup, or extract.
5. If frozen solid, place in microwave for 30 seconds, to thaw, before serving.

• *1/2 cup cottage cheese or 1 cup yogurt*
• *2 ozs. pineapple* • *4 ozs. strawberries*
• *sugar-free Da Vinci coconut or coffee syrup or Frontier coconut flavoring*

Serving amount: 6 ozs. fruit, 1 dairy or protein

Fruit with Dairy/Protein

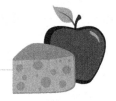

Tofu Key Lime Pie-Pudding

1. Put the tofu, ricotta cheese, and unsweetened soymilk into a food processor; process until the mixture is smooth and creamy.
2. Pour the lime juice into a small saucepan and stir in the gelatin; allow to stand for about 3 to 5 minutes to soften the gelatin.
3. Stir the mixture over low heat until the gelatin is dissolved, about 2 minutes.
4. Stir in the tofu-ricotta cheese mixture.
5. Pour the filling into the completely cooled crust. Refrigerate until the filling is firm, about 2 to 3 hours, before serving. Makes 5 portions. Each portion equals 1 protein, 1 oz. fruit

---

- *1 cup unsweetened soymilk*
- *1 1/2 cups mashed silken firm tofu (12 ozs.)*
- *1 cup nonfat ricotta cheese*
- *sweetener (optional)*
- *6 ozs. freshly squeezed Key lime juice (juice from about 9 Key limes)*
- *1 envelope (1 tb.) unflavored gelatin*
- *garnish (optional lime slices*

Serving amount: 1 oz. fruit, 1 protein

Tofu Strawberry Smoothie

1. Blend the tofu and cleaned and washed fresh strawberries in a blender or with a hand mixer.
2. Chill before drinking. Or slightly freeze or churn in frozen ice cream-yogurt maker.

- *4 ozs. mashed silken firm tofu*
- *1/2 cup cold water*
- *6 ozs. fresh strawberries*

Serving amount: 6 ozs. fruit, 1/2 or 2 ozs. protein, 1 cup dairy

Fruit with Dairy/Protein

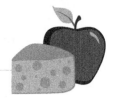

Turkey & Cranberry Relish (Separate)

1. Cranberry Sauce (no sugar) recipe.
2. Serve with turkey.

• *4 ozs. turkey* • *6 ozs. homemade cranberry sauce (no sugar)*

Serving amount: 6 ozs. fruit, 4 ozs. protein

Turkey Salad - Cape Cod Cranberry Style

1. Mince the raw cranberries and orange:
A 12 or 16 ozs. bag of raw cranberries & 1 orange equals (3) single portions of fruit.
2. Divide the cranberry relish into 3 portions.
3. Set aside.
4. Use one portion of the cranberry relish for a single serving of Cape Cod Turkey Salad. Or use all 3 portions if making all 12 ozs. of the cooked turkey.
5. Option to freeze.
6. Mix the cold cooked turkey, the mayonnaise, and the celery.
7. Add the raw cranberry relish to the turkey salad for Cape Cod Turkey Salad.

• *1 serving cranberry relish*
• *4 ozs. chopped cooked turkey*
• *1 tbs. mayonnaise* • *1/2 cup celery*

Serving amount: 6 ozs. fruit, 4 ozs. protein, 1 tbs. oil

Yogurt - Strained with Fruit

1. Take a coffee filter or a large piece of cheesecloth.
2. Measure 1 cup of plain yogurt.
3. Place the yogurt in the filter or cheesecloth.
4. Suspend the filter or cheesecloth over a bowl overnight, so it may strain out the liquid.
5. Add 6 ozs fruit for breakfast or a before-bedtime metabolic.

• *1 cup yogurt* • *6 ozs. fruit*

Serving amount: 6 ozs. fruit, 1 protein or dairy

Fruit with Protein with Starch/Grain

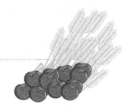

Apple Oat Bran Muffins- Muffins I

1. Combine ingredients.
2. Fill muffin cups sprayed with non-aerosol oil mist.
3. Heat oven to 325 degrees.
4. Bake muffins for 20-30 minutes.
5. See if a knife or fork placed in the center of a muffin comes out clean, to test if they are done. Makes 1 portion.

- *1 beaten egg • 2 egg whites • 1/2 cup oat bran*
- *1/2 cup cottage cheese • 6 ozs. grated apple*
- *1/4 tsp. cinnamon • 1/8 tsp. baking soda*
- *sweetener (optional)*

Serving amount: 6 ozs. fruit, 4 ozs. protein, 1 cup dairy, 1 cup cooked starch/grain

Apple & Oatmeal Cooked

1. Chop apple.
2. Add apple to cooked oatmeal.
3. Use large microwavable bowl as oatmeal will steam upward during cooking.
4. Add spices. 6. Put 1/2 cup milk, cooked oatmeal and apple with 1/2 cup water in bowl.
5. Cook in microwave for 5 minutes. Or cook in slow cooker for 15-20 minutes.

- *1 apple • 1 cup milk • 2 ozs. dry oatmeal*

Serving amount: 6 ozs. fruit, 1 cup dairy, 1 cup cooked starch/grain

Blueberry Oat Buttermilk Crepe- Crepe I

1. Mix ingredients.
2. Cook on each side in a frying pan or in a saute pan.
3. Top with fruit.
4. Serve.

- *1 cup buttermilk • 1/2 cup dry oat bran or oatmeal • 6 ozs. fresh blueberries • 2 beaten eggs • 1 tsp. oil*

Serving amount: 6 ozs. fruit, 1 cup dairy, 1 protein, 1 cup cooked starch/grain, 1 tsp. oil

Blueberry Oat Muffins - Muffin II

1. Mix well.
2. Pour into small round container, diameter 3 inches.
3. Microwave on high 3-4 minutes.
4. Let cool 2 minutes. 5. Turn onto plate.

- *2 ozs. oat bran • 1 egg • 2 oz fruit*
- *blueberries ~ pineapple or a apple*
- *3/4 tsp. cinnamon*
- *non-alcohol vanilla flavoring to taste*

Serving amount: 1/3 fruit, 1/2 protein, 1 cup cooked starch/grain

Fruit with Protein with Starch/Grain

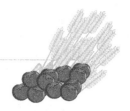

Blueberry Muffins or Loaf - Muffins III

1. Beat eggs.
2. Mix remaining ingredients into eggs.
3. Heat oven to 325 degrees.
4. Pour mixture into a small muffin tins, about half full, or small loaf pan sprayed with non-aerosol non-fat cooking spray.
5. Bake for 20-30 minutes.
6. Let cool for 5 minutes.
 Variations: Use 6 ounces chopped peaches, pear, apple, or pineapple in place of blueberries. Makes 1 portion.

• *2 eggs or 4 egg whites* • *1/2 cup dry oatmeal or oat bran* • *1/3 cup powdered milk or 1/2 cup cottage cheese* • *1/4 tsp. cinnamon* • *6 ozs. blueberries* • *1/8 tsp. baking soda* • *sweetener (optional)* • *Swedish seasoning with vanilla and cardamon or cinnamon and nutmeg (see Swedish Spice Blend in Recipes)*

Serving amount: 6 ozs. fruit, 4 ozs. protein or dairy-free protein, 1 cup dairy, 1 cup cooked starch/grain

Cranberry Brown Rice Pudding I

1. Mix egg with milk, rice, cinnamon and nutmeg.
2. Pour mixture into the small glass baking dish or loaf pan.
3. Place the glass fish or loaf pan in a shallow cooking dish filled with 1/2 inch water.
4. Pre-heat oven to 325 degrees.
6. Oven Bake - 325 degrees - estimated cooking time 25 minutes. Microwave - on High - estimated cooking time 6 minutes, or until liquid is absorbed.

• *1/2 cup cooked brown rice* • *1 egg* • *1 cup milk* • *1/4 tsp. cinnamon* • *1/4 tsp. nutmeg* • *6 ozs. cranberry sauce or relish (homemade - no sugar)* • *sweetener (optional)*

Serving amount: 1 protein, 1 dairy, 1/2 cup cooked starch/grain. Variations: Use 6 ounces chopped peaches, pear, apple, or pineapple in place of cranberries. Makes 1 portion.

Fruit with Protein with Starch/Grain

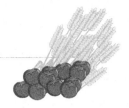

Lime Pudding or Cheesecake

1. Put wet ingredients into a blender and blend.
2. For zest, take lime and grate 1 tbs. peel into blended mixture. A zester utensil, with the flat blade with a beveled end and 5 small holes, will create curly zest from the lime peel. Zest is colorful and flavorful.
3. For crust blend 2 ozs. oat bran and 1 egg white. Roll pie crust blend into a small ball then into a disk. Mist muffin tins or loan pan or pie plate with non-aerosol oil mist. Press crust into muffin tins, a small loaf pan or a pie plate or small tart plates.
4. Bake crusts for 5-10 minutes at 325 degrees in oven or roaster oven or for 1-2 minutes in microwave. If using a microwave, make sure muffin tins or loaf pan or pie plate are not metal.
5. Pour filling blend into muffin tins, loaf pan or pie plate. Refrigerate for 1 hour. Top with Lime Peel or Mint Sprig. Makes 4 portions. Each portion equals 1 protein: 3 ozs. tofu & 1/3 egg white, 1/4 tbs. soynut butter; 1/4 cup cooked starch/grain, 6 ozs. fruit.

- *1 1/2 cups or 12 ozs. silken tofu*
- *sweetener (optional)* • *1 tbs. no alcohol lemon flavoring   1 tsp. no alcohol vanilla flavoring*
- *1 tbs. lime zest* • *1/2 cup lime juice or juice of 2 limes* • *1 tbs. unsweetened soynut butter (optional)* • *2 oz. dry oat bran* • *1 egg white*
- *non-aerosol oil mist*

Serving amount: 6 ozs. fruit, 1 protein, 1/4 cup cooked starch/grain

Oat Bran Muffins or Loaf - Muffins IV

1. Use a small loaf pan sprayed with non-aerosol oil mist.
2. Preheat oven to 325 degrees.
3. Mix ingredients and pour into loaf pan.
4. Cook 20-25 minutes.
5. Check by inserting a knife into the middle of the loaf. Knife will come out clean when the loaf is done.

- *2 eggs* • *1/3 cup non-fat powdered milk or 1/2 cup cottage cheese* • *1/4 tsp. cinnamon*
- *1/2 cup oat bran* • *6 ozs. diced fruit*
- *sweetener ((optional)*

Serving amount: 6 ozs. fruit, 1 protein, 1 cup dairy, 1 cup cooked starch/grain

Fruit with Protein with Starch/Grain

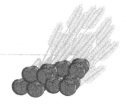

Oat Bran Waffle with Fruit

1. Mix oat bran, oil, dry milk to eggs.
2. Heat your waffle maker and non-aerosol non-fat cooking spray.
3. Spoon mixture onto waffle maker. Spread smoothly.
4. Cook according to the directions of your waffle maker.
5. Spoon 6 ozs. chopped stewed fruit (strawberries & rhubard) or chopped fresh fruit on top.
6. Waffles can be cooked then frozen.
7. When ready to use, you can reheat waffles in a toaster oven or microwave.

- *2 eggs well beaten in large bowl*
- *1/3 cup non-fat powdered milk*
- *6 ozs. fresh fruit • 2 ozs. dry oat bran*
- *non-fat cooking spray • 1 tsp. oil*
- *sweetener (optional) • 1/2 tsp. cinnamon*

Serving amount: 6 ozs. fruit, 4 ozs protein, 1 cup dairy, 1 cup cooked starch/grain,

Oatmeal - Hot Apple Chunks or Blueberries - Dairy-Free Soymilk

1. Peel, core, and slice apple. If using blueberries, rinse the blueberries. Weigh 6 ozs. apple or 1/2 cup blueberries.
2. In a saucepan, microwaveable bowl, or slow cooker, place the oats, the water, the sliced apple or the blueberries, and the spices.
3. Cook. Saucepan - on High - estimated cooking time - 10 minutes. Microwave - on High - estimated cooking time 5 minutes. Slow Cooker - on High - estimated cooking time - 20 minutes. Whole oatmeal will cook faster than sleel cut oats. Steel cut oats will cook up soft if you let it cook longer. The longer you let it cook, the thicker the consistency will be.

- *6 ozs. apple or 1/2 cup blueberries*
- *1 cup lowfat milk or unsweetened soymilk*
- *2 ozs. dry whole oatmeal*
- *1/2 tsp. cinnamon*
- *1/2 tsp. nutmeg • 8 ozs. unsweetened soymilk*

Serving amount: 6 ozs. fruit, 1 cup dairy, 1 cup cooked starch/grain

Fruit with Protein with Starch/Grain

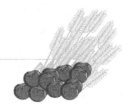

Peach or Other Fruit - Yogurt-Grain Cooked Combo

1. Mix the peaches and yogurt together in a small serving bowl. In another bowl, mix together the oat bran pancake ingredients.
2. Pour the oat bran pancake mixture into a small flat bottom pan sprayed with non-aerosol oil mist.
3. Microwave pancake for 3-4 minutes until the pancake is formed. Slide it on to your yogurt and fruit mixture.

- *6 ozs. peaches or any other fruit you like*
- *1 cup plain yogurt*
- *oat bran pancake: 1 oz. oat bran with 1/4 club soda or water*

Serving amount: 6 ozs. fruit, 1 protein or 1 dairy, 1/2 cup cooked starch/grain

Pear Muffins or Loaf - Dairy-Free Muffin V

1. Mix all ingredients well.
2. Heat oven to 325 degrees.
3. Spray muffin tin or small loaf pan with cooking spray. 4. Fill each tin or loaf half full.
5. Cook for 15-20 minutes or until the knife comes out dry.

- *2 large eggs or 4 egg whites • 1/4 tsp. nutmeg*
- *1 cup cooked grain, brown rice, oatmeal or millet • 1/4 tsp. cinnamon • 6 ozs. chopped pears*
- *sweetener (optional)*

Serving amount: 6 ozs. fruit, 1 protein or dairy-free substitute, 1 cup cooked starch/grain

Pear Oat Bran Baked Pudding

1. Preheat oven to 325 degrees.
2. Mix well eggs, oat bran, pear and cottage cheese in bowl, adding sweetener (optional).
3. Dissolve contents of plain no-calorie gelatin packet into hot water.
4. Add to egg mixture.
5. Pour mixture into glass pie plate sprayed with non-aerosol non-fat cooking spray.
6. Sprinkle with cinnamon and bake for 20-30 minutes. Makes 1 portion.

- *2 eggs • 1/2 cup dry oat bran • 6 ozs. pear sliced, with or without peel • 1/2 cup low fat cottage cheese • 1 packet gelatin • 1/4 cup hot water • sweetener (optional) • 1/2 tsp. cinnamon*

Serving amount: 6 ozs. fruit, 4 ozs. protein or dairy-free substitute, 1 cup dairy or dairy-free substitute, 1 cup cooked starch/grain

Fruit with Protein with Starch/Grain

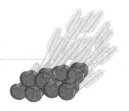

Pineapple - Blueberry Ricotta or Cottage Cheese Crepe - Crepe II

1. Weigh the fruit serving (1/2 cup serving or 1/4 cup of pineapple & blueberries each).
2. Separate into two 3 ozs portions.
3. Blend, mash, or whip together the fruit, cottage cheese and egg.
4. Use a pump spray cooking oil to oil the saute pan or griddle.
5. Drop the batter onto the saute pan. Brown on both sides.
6. Place the remaining 3 ozs of fruit on top of the crepe. Serve & Eat.

- *6 ozs. blueberries or pineapple*
- *1/4 cup or 2 ozs. ricotta or cottage cheese*
- *1 raw egg • 1 tsp oil*

Serving amount: 6 ozs. fruit, 1 dairy or protein

Pineapple Crushed - Coconut Flavor Brown Rice Pudding II

1. In a large, heavy saucepan, heat the crushed pineapple and coconut flavoring, 2 teaspoons cinnamon (make sure it doesn't clump up), salt, and cooked brown rice.
2. Add the unsweetened soymilk. Immediately reduce the heat to low. Simmer until the brown rice is very tender.
3. Give the mixture a good stir, and let the pudding sit, uncovered, for a few minutes to cool and thicken slightly.

- *1/2 cup crushed pineapple*
- *1 cup cooked brown rice*
- *1 tsp. non-alcohol coconut flavoring*
- *1 /2 cup unsweetened soymilk*

Serving amount: 1. fruit, 1/2 dairy or protein, 1 cup cooked starch/grain

Protein-Grain Fruit Breakfasts - Dairy-Free

1. Prepare each breakfast combination for: 1 fruit, 1 dairy-free substitute, 1 protein, starch-grain.

- *6 ozs. fruit, 4 scrambled egg whites or 4 oz. tofu, grain, 1 cup cooked starch/grain*
- *Shakes made with 6 ozs. fruit, 1 cup unsweetened soymilk, protein, and grain.*
- *6 ozs. fruit, 4 ozs. salmon, 1 cup cooked brown rice*

Serving amount: 6 ozs. fruit, 1 protein, 1 cup cooked starch/grain

Fruit with Protein with Starch/Grain

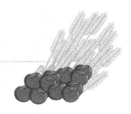

Strained Yogurt Oatmeal Fruit-Filled Crepes - Crepe III

1. A day ahead prepare strained yogurt.
2. Put 1 cup yogurt into a paper coffee filter and place filled paper filter in a strainer or colander over a bowl to drain. You may also use cheesecloth to strain the yogurt.
3. Place the draining yogurt in the refrigerator.
4. Mix together eggs, oats, water and spices.
5. Cook crepe in preheated non-stick pan on medium high.
6. Turn crepe to brown other side.
7. After you slip the crepe onto a plate, fill the crepe with the strained yogurt and fruit.
8. Roll up crepe.
9. Cool slightly.
10. Serve.

- *1/2 cup crushed no juice pineapple, blueberries, or 6 ozs. minced strawberries or finely chopped apple*
- *2 tbs. water*
- *2 eggs* • *1 cup strained yogurt*
- *2 ozs. dry oatmeal* • *cinnamon, nutmeg, vanilla (optional)*

Serving amount: 6 ozs. fruit, 1 protein, 1 cup dairy, 1 cup cooked starch/grain

Dairy/Protein & Dairy-Free Substitutes

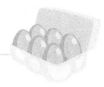

Chai Spiced Iced or Hot Tea

1. In a medium saucepan,
bring the milk just to boil.
2. Stir in the remaining ingredients
except for the carbonated water.
3. Reduce heat to low and
simmer, uncovered, for 3 minutes.
4. Remove the tea bags and strain; chill.
5. Serve over ice, adding an equal amount of
the carbonated water to each serving. This
tea is also terrific when served warm in mugs
- just replace the carbonated water with warm
water.

- *2 cups skim milk • sweetener (optional)*
- *1/2 tsp. ground cinnamon*
- *1/4 tsp. ground ginger*
- *1/8 tsp. allspice*
- *4 tea bags*
- *2 cups chilled, unflavored, unsweetened
carbonated water*

Serving amount: 1 protein or dairy

Cheesecake - Italian Style with Ricotta Cheese

1. Preheat oven to 350 degrees.
2. With a food processor, grind dry oatmeal
until fine.
3. With food processor or mixer mix finely
ground oatmeal or oat bran, sweetener
(optional) and cinnamon together. Add
vanilla and cream soda. The mixture will
turn into the consistency of play dough.
4. Divide mixture by 6, and with your hands,
form into balls and then flatten into small
disks.
5. Thoroughly coat a mini 6 muffin or 6
mini-loaf pan with non-aerosol oil mist.
6. Place the discs in the center of each of the
muffin molds and line and shape with your
fingers into the bottom crust.
7. In the food processor, combine yogurt
(labne), ricotta cheese, egg, lemon peel,
remaining sweetener (optional) and lemon
flavors..
8. Mix well.

- *48 ozs. strained yogurt or labne • 8 ozs. ricotta
cheese • 4 eggs • 2 tbs. + 2 tsp. lemon flavor*
- *2 tbs. + 2 tsp. lemon peel • sweetener (optional)*
- *6 ozs. rolled oatmeal, ground fine • 2-4 tbs.
water • 2 tbs. + 2 tsp. non-alcohol vanilla extract.
Makes 6 portions. Each portion equals 1 protein,
8 ozs. or 1 cup dairy, 1 ozs. starch/grain*

Serving amount: 1 protein, 8 ozs. or 1 cup
dairy, 1 ozs. or 1/2 cup cooked starch/grain

Dairy/Protein & Dairy-Free Substitutes

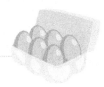

Coconut Custard

1. Combine ingredients and put in loaf pan or ramekin. Bake 450 for 15 minutes.
2. Reduce oven to 325 and cook for 35 minutes or until knife comes out clean.
3. Cool in fridge. May be eaten warm or cool.

• *1 egg* • *8 ozs. milk, mix with sweetener (optional)* • *vanilla extract* • *coconut extract (alcohol free extracts - like Frontier)* • *salt (pinch to pull out sweet).*

Serving amount: 1 cup dairy, 1/2 protein

Coffee Crunch Ice Cream

1. Mix in bowl.
2. Then add to ice cream maker.
3. Let ice cream maker run for 20 minutes.
4. Or mix in blender. Pour into ice cube tray or flat bowl. Freeze. Makes 2 portions. Each portion equals 1 cup dairy/protein,

---

• *1 cup plain yogurt, 3/4 cup milk*
• *1 ozs. soy nuts* • *1 tbs. any alcohol-free flavor extract (like Frontier)* • *1 tbs. instant coffee*

Serving amount: 1 cup dairy/protein

Coffee Ice Cream

1. Mix in bowl then add to ice cream maker.
2. Mix for 20 minutes depends on brand of machine.

• *4 ozs. plain yogurt* • *8 ozs. milk* • *1 tbs. instant coffee* • *1 tbs. maple no alcohol extract (like Frontier)* • *sweetener (optional)*

Serving amount: 1 cup dairy, 4 ozs. or 1/2 cup or 4 ozs. protein

Coffee Shakes

1. Blend a lot starting on low setting and working way up to the highest setting.
2. Let it get really airy and frothy...!!! It really seems like there is milk in it, but there isn't!
3. Some people keep brewed de-cafe in the fridge in pourable containers. Some people use instant coffee.

• *black coffee, already brewed or instant crystals*
• *ice, sweetener (optional)* • *alcohol-free extracts like Frontier*

Serving amount: water used

Dairy/Protein & Dairy-Free Substitutes

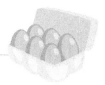

Cottage Cheese Crepe - Crepe IV

1. Mix all ingredients.
2. Heat a saute pan.
3. Brown on both sides and serve.

• *1/2 cup cottage cheese* • *1 tsp. oil*
• *2 eggs*

Serving: 1 dairy, 1 protein, 1 tsp. non-aerosol oil mist mist

Dairy-Free Substitutes - Proteins

1. Prepare each dairy-free protein and use as a dairy-free substitute or a protein.

Each of these is a complete dairy or dairy-free substitute or protein:
• *4 scrambled egg whites*
• *4 ozs. tofu*
• *1 cup unsweetened soymilk*
• *2 ozs. soynut butter (unsweetened)*

Serving amount: 1 protein or dairy

Egg Custard

1. Whisk together eggs, milk, spices.
2. Pour into 2 individual 1 cup oven proof pyrex glass bowls. Sprinkle with nutmeg.
3. Put bowls in a cake pan and pour boiling water around the bowls to about 1 inch from top of bowls.
4. Bake at 350 degrees for 35 minutes or until firm. Makes 2 portions. Each portion equals 1 protein and 1 cup dairy.

• *4 eggs beaten* • *2 cups of scalded fat-free milk*
• *sweetener (optional)* • *1 tsp. no alcohol vanilla flavoring, nutmeg*

Serving amount: 1 dairy, 1 protein

Egg Custard - Coconut-Flavored

1. Mix in aluminum loaf pan or ramekin.
2. Bake 450 for 15 minutes Reduce oven to 325, and cook for 35 minutes, or until knife comes out clean. Cool in fridge. Add fruit on top if serving at breakfast.

• *1 egg* • *1 cup milk* • *alcohol-free coconut flavoring, maple flavoring or coffee flavoring*
• *sweetener (optional)* • *pinch of salt to bring out the sweet flavor. Makes 1 portion.*

Serving amount: 1/2 protein, 1 cup dairy

Dairy/Protein & Dairy-Free Substitutes

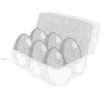

Farmer Cheese Omelet

1. Spray bottom of large fry pan with non-aerosol oil mist and heat it.
2. Pour eggs into the pan and let cook.
3. Spread and smear farmer cheese all over evenly and let cook a bit more until it looks blended.
4. Fold over the eggs and cheese into an omelet so the outside is browned and crisp. Flip.
5. Slice into appropriate single serving. For breakfast, add warm berries or other fruit on top. Makes 2 portions. Each portion equals 1 protein, 1 dairy.

• *4 whipped eggs* • *4 ozs. farmer cheese, creamy kind (or large curd whole milk cottage cheese)* • *non-aerosol oil mist* • *cinnamon if you like it (or extract if you want it sweet). Makes 2 portions.*

Serving amount: 1 protein, 1 dairy

Lemon Custard, Baked

1. Beat ingredients together in a bowl.
2. Place custard cups in a baking pan and fill.
3. Pour boiling water around custard cups.
4. Bake at 350 for one hour; allow to cool before serving.

• *8 ozs. milk* • *1 egg* • *1 tsp. lemon flavoring*
• *sweetener (optional)* • *1 tsp. nutmeg*
• *1 tsp. lemon peel* • *variation: 1 tsp. cinnamon*

Serving amount: 8 ozs. or 1 cup dairy, 1/2 protein or 1 egg

Soy Milk, How To Make

1. Rinse and soak the beans overnight (or at least 10 hours) in the fridge.
2. When ready, drain and rinse. Either grind the beans into a paste using a grain mill and add to a pot of 12 cups boiling water OR process the beans in a blender or food processor with boiling water (3/4 cup beans to 1 3/4 cup boiling water at a time) and pour into a big heavy pot. (Note: It is important to not over estimate your blenders abilities. Be careful to not burn out your blender while grinding beans. A food processor offers better results (with sharp blade)).
3. Bring this mixture to a boil stirring over medium to high heat.
4. Turn down immediately after it starts to boil, or you'll have a mess. Now let it simmer (no stirring necessary) for 20-30 minutes.
5. Meanwhile, line a colander with a thin cloth, and set it up over a big bowl or another pot. Ladle the cooked soymilk into the colander, straining the pulp (called okara) in the cloth and allowing the milk to collect in the bowl. You may add more water, sweetener, vanilla extract, or sea salt. The pulp okara can be steamed for an hour and used as a soy protein like tofu. Measure soy protein at 4 ozs. protein or unsweetened soy milk as 1 cup dairy. Makes a gallon or so.

• *2 cups of dried soy beans* • *water*

Serving amount: 8 ozs. or 1 cup dairy or portein

— 77 —

Dairy/Protein & Dairy-Free Substitutes

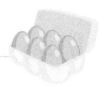

Tofu Scrambled with Herbs

1. Beat ingredients together in a bowl.
2. Spray frying pan with non-aerosol oil mist, or prepare microwavable bowl
3. Scramble tofu with herbs in the frying pan, or beat the scrambled tofu with herbs and cook in microwave for 3 minutes.

• *4 ozs. firm tofu* • *1/2 tsp. garlic salt* • *1 tsp. lonion flakes* • *1 tsp. dill or rosemary*

Serving amount: 1 protein

Tofu Vanilla Maple Custard

1. Put ingredients in a blender. Blend.
2. Pour blended mixture into 4 cups. Refrigerate for 1 hour. Makes 4 portions. Each portion equals 4 ozs. tofu or 1 protein or 1 dairy.

• *4 ozs. silken tofu* • *1 tsp. vanilla flavoring* • *1 tsp. maple flavoring*

Serving amount: 1 dairy or 1 protein

Yogurt I - Homemade - No Machine Make It Yourself Yogurt - Requires Cooking Thermometer

1. Mix powdered milk and water.
2. Heat carefully, watching all the time witha cooking thermometer, to 180 degrees. Stirthe heating milk so it does not stick to thebottom.
3. Remove from heat and watch the cooking-thermometer until the milk cools down to 100 degrees.
4. Stir in the yogurt starter.
5. Pour mix into a or large heavy glass.
6. Wrap the jar in towels. Put a towel aroundthe top of the jar.
7. Place the har into a softsided thermal bagor hard sided thermal cooler. Be sure toinclude the towels wrapped around the jar.
8. Close lid.
9. The heat from the mixture will beretained and culture the yogurt until it is set.
The Yogurt will be done in 8 to 10 hours.

• *1 1/3 c powdered dry skim milk* • *4 cups water*
• *1/2 cup live culture yogurt for starter*

Serving: 1 protein or dairy

Dairy/Protein & Dairy-Free Substitutes

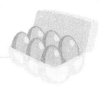

Yogurt II - Strained Greek Yogurt

1. Measure one cup yogurt before straining.
2. Strain 1 cup of yogurt overnight
in astrainer lined with a coffee filter.
3. Place strainer over a bowl and
refrigerateovernight.

• *1 cup or 8 ozs. yogurt*

Serving amount: 1 dairy or 1 protein

Yogurt III - Homemade - with Electric Yogurtmaker

1. To make cost-saving homemade
yogurt,invest in an electric yogurtmaker.
Makes 4 portions. Each portion equals 1 cup
yogurt or 1 protein or 1 dairy.

• *1 1/3 c powdered dry skim milk* • *4 cups water*
• *1/2 cup live culture yogurt for starter*

Serving: 1 protein or dairy

Protein - Animal & Soy

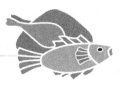

Beef, Cajun Prime Rib

1. Place the roast, standing on the rib bones, in a very large roasting pan.
2. Then make several dozen punctures through the silver skin so seasoning can permeate the meat.
3. Pour a very generous, even layer of black pepper over the top of the meat until evenly covered; repeat procedure with garlic powder, then salt.
4. Refrigerate 24 hours. Bake ribs in a 550 oven until fat is brown and crispy, about 35 minutes. Remove from oven and cool slightly.
5. Refrigerate until very well chilled, about 3 hours.
6. Scrape off seasonings, then slice between ribs into 6 steaks; trim the cooked surface from the two pieces that were on the end.
7. Coat with seasoning mix and blacken in a cast-iron skillet, or grill.

• *seasoning mix: 1 tb. + 2 tsp. salt*
• *1 tb. + 2 tsp. white pepper • 1 tb. + 2 tsp. whole fennel seeds • 1 tb. + 3/4 tsp. black pepper*
• *2 1/2 tsp. dry mustard • 2 1/2 tsp. cayenne, roast: 1 (4-bone) prime rib of beef roast about 10 1/2 lbs • 1/4 cup black pepper • 1/4 cup garlic powder • 1/4 cup salt*

Serving amount: 4 ozs. protein

Beef, Pork or Lamb Keftadhes

1. Mix together all ingredients. 2. Shape into patties or meatballs. 3. Place on baking sheet and bake in preheated 350° oven for about 30 minutes or until brown.

• *2 lbs. ground meat • 2 tbs. onion flakes • 2 tbs. parsley flakes • 1 tsp. chopped mint • 1 tsp. oregano*

Serving amount: 4 ozs. protein, non-aerosol oil mist

Beef, Savory Meatballs

1. Heat oven to 350°F.
2. In a mixing bowl, combine sirloin, oat bran, parsley and seasoning. If necessary, add a little water to beef mixture to hold it together.
3. Roll into meat balls.
4. Place on an broiling rack, sprayed with zero-calorie butter spray, and bake 15 minutes.

• *4 ozs. sirloin • 1/8 cup oat bran*
• *abstinent Italian or pizza seasoning*
• *non-aerosol oil mist*

Serving amount: 4 ozs. protein

Protein - Animal & Soy

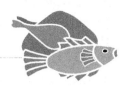

Beef Grilled with Lemongrass

1. Combine soy sauce, oil, vinegar, lemongrass, garlic, red pepper flakes, mint leaves, and sweetener in a blender or food-processor and purée the hell out of them.
2. Transfer into a shallow baking dish.
3. Thread the beef onto skewers and add to the marinade.
4. Refrigerate at least 2-4 hours, turning once.
5. Preheat the grill or broiler, very hot.
6. Grill skewers for 2 to 3 minutes on each side.

• *2 tbs. soy sauce or Bragg's Amino Acids (tastes like soy sauce only with less sodium)*
• *1 tb. white vinegar • 2 1/2 tbs. minced fresh lemongrass • 1 tb. peanut oil • 2 cloves garlic pressed • 1 tsp. red pepper flakes • 1/4 cup fresh mint leaves • 1 tsp. sweetener (optional)*
• *1 1/2 lbs beef, sliced into thin strips*

Serving amount: 4 ozs. protein

Beef Kofta Curry

1. For koftas, fry onion powder, ginger, and garlic in zero calorie cooking spray until brown. (Or you may use ground ginger and garlic powder to mix with the meat.)
2. Add to remaining kofta ingredients, mix well, and mold into balls 2 inches in diameter.
3. For sauce, grind garlic and ginger to a paste in blender or food processor.
4. Fry onion flakes mix and garlic/ginger paste in zero calorie cooking spray until light brown.
5. Add tomato sauce, 3 cups water, salt, and cayenne.
6. Bring to a boil.
7. Add koftas and cook, uncovered, until all the water evaporates.
8. Gently fold in garam masala.

• *koftas sauce • 1 pound ground beef*
• *3 tbs. onion flakes • 1 tb. onion powder*
• *1 clove garlic • 4 cloves garlic pressed*
• *2 inches ginger peeled*
• *1 inch ginger, grated • 4 tbs. tomato sauce*
• *salt to taste • 2 tsp. garam masala*
• *1/4 tsp. cayenne*

Serving amount: 4 ozs protein. 1/8 cup

Protein - Animal & Soy

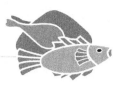

Beef or Turkey or Lamb Meatball Paprikash

1. Combine pork, veal, or pork or lamb alone,salt, onion powder, and fennel seeds in a large bowl or food processor; blend well.
2. Shape into 1 1/2" balls.
3. Heat oil in 12" skillet over medium-high heat;
4. Add meatballs and cook about 12 minutes, turning frequently until well browned on all sides.
5. Using a slotted spoon, remove meatballs to plate.
6. Add paprika, tomato paste, and about 1/2 cup water, and stir to mix well.
7. Increase heat to high; bring to a boil.
8. Return meatballs to pan.
9. Reduce heat and simmer, covered, for 10 minutes, until meatballs are cooked through.
10. Uncover and stir soy milk into meatball mixture.
11.Cook gently until sauce thickens. Makes 5 portions. Each portion equals 4 ozs. protein.

• *1 lb. combined ground beef or turkey or lamb*
• *1 tb. fennel seeds • 1 tsp. salt • 2 tbs. vegetable oil • 1 tb. onion powder • 2 tbs. paprika • 2 tbs. tomato paste • 1 cup soy milk • 2 tbs. chopped fresh parsley*

Serving amount: 4 ozs. protein

Beef Roast or Chunks - Broiled, Grilled as Kabobs or Roasted with Seasonings

1. Take small beef roast.
2. Put in a pan.
3. Put pan in a 350 degree oven.
4. Roast about 30-45 minutes until no longer pink.
5. Pieces of beef may be cut and placed on skewers and grilled as kabobs. Makes 4 portions. Each portion equals 4 ozs. protein.

• *1 lb. beef • salt • 6 cloves garlic, coarsely chopped • 1 clove garlic, pressed • 1 tb. minced parsley • May be cooked and eaten plan with salt and pepper only.*

Serving amount: 4 ozs. protein

Protein - Animal & Soy

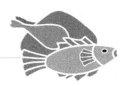

Beef Roasted Louisiana Style

1. Combine onion flakes and seasonings in a small bowl with 2 Tb water; mix well.
2. Place the roast in a large roasting pan, fat side up. With a large knife make 6-12 deep slits in the meat, down to a depth of about 1/2 inch from the bottom; do not cut all the way through.
3. Fill the pockets with the seasoning mixture, reserving 1 Tb to rup over the top of the roast.
4. Bake uncovered at 300 until a meat thermometer reads 160 for medium doneness, about 3 hours.

- *2 tbs. onion powder • 2 tbs. onion flakes*
- *1 tsp. salt • 1 tsp. white pepper*
- *3/4 tsp. black pepper • 3/4 tsp. minced garlic*
- *1/2 tsp. dry mustard • 1/2 tsp. cayenne*
- *1 (3 1/2-4 lb) boneless sirloin roast or top round roast.*

Serving amount: 4 ozs. protein

Beef Slices with Rosemary

1. Heat a large heavy frying pan and add non-aerosol oil mist and garlic.
2. Pan-fry the meat on both sides quickly over medium-high heat.
3. Salt and pepper the meat and remove it to a heated serving platter.
4. Add the rosemary to the pan along with 1/4 cup water.
5. Deglaze the pan and pour the resulting sauce over the meat. Makes 4 portions. Each portion equals 4 ozs protein, non-aerosol oil mist.

- *non-aerosol oil mist • 2 cloves garlic, coarsely chopped • 1 lb. lean roast beef sliced quite thin*
- *salt and freshly ground black pepper to taste*
- *1 tb. chopped fresh rosemary*

Serving amount: 4 ozs. protein, non-aerosol oil mist

Protein - Animal & Soy

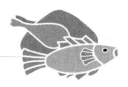

Beef Tenderloin

1. Combine everything but the meat in a small bowl. 2. Line a baking pan with foiland place the roast on it. 3. Spread the sauceover the roast, covering it as thoroughly as possible. 4. Broil at 500 degreesfor 30-35 minutes.

• 1 beef tenderloin, beef roast, london broil, etc • 2-4 cloves garlic, pressed • salt • 2 tbs. mustard • 1 tb.parsley • 2 tbs. basil • 2 tbs. marjoram • 2 tbs. thyme • ground pepper • non-aerosol oil mist

Serving amount: 4 ozs. protein, non-aerosol oil mist

Catfish or Tilapia - Baked with Mock Sour Cream

1. Preheat oven to 350 degrees.
2. Prepare a baking dish by spraying it with non-aerosol oil mist.
3. Rinse the fillets in water and then dry between layers of paper towels.
4. Arrange the fillets in the baking dish.
5. In a small bowl, combine the mock sour cream, yogurt, vinegar, paprika, pepper, and thyme;
6. Spread the mixture over the fish and sprinkle with dill.
7. Bake for 15 minutes, or until the fish flakes pen touched with a fork.
8. Garnish with lemon wedges and parsley, if desired. Makes 4 portions. Each portion equals 4 ozs. protein, 1 oz. or 1/8 cup dairy

• 1 pound (16 ozs.) catfish fillets • 2 tsp. mock sour cream • 1/2 cup plain nonfat yogurt • 1/2 tsp. vinegar • 1/2 tsp. ground celery seed • 1/4 tsp. paprika • 1/4 tsp. freshly ground white or black pepper • 1/4 tsp. thyme • 1 tsp. fresh dill (or a pinch of dried dill per fillet) • 1 lemon, cut into 4 wedges (optional) • Fresh chopped or dried parsley (optional).

Serving amount: 4 ozs. protein, 1 oz. or 1/8 cup dairy, non-aerosol oil mist

Catfish with Oat Bran Crumbled Coating

1. Preheat oven to 350 degrees.
2. Prepare a baking dish by spraying it with non-aerosol oil mist.
3. Rinse the fillets in water. Leave wet.
4. On a large plate dip the fillets in 1 ozs. dry oat bran.
5. Arrange the fillets in the baking dish.
6. Bake for 15-20 minutes, or until the fish flakes pen touched with a fork.
7. Garnish with lemon wedges and parsley, if desired. Makes 4 portions. Each portion equals 4 ozs. protein, 1/4 ozs. starch/grain

---

• 1 pound (16 ozs.) catfish fillets • 1 ozs. dry oat bran flakes • 1 lemon, cut into 4 wedges (optional) • Fresh chopped or dried parsley (optional)

Serving amount: 4 ozs. protein, 1/4 ozs. starch/grain, non-aerosol oil mist

Protein - Animal & Soy

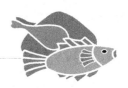

Ceviche Seafood Salad with Lime Zest

1. Clean and cook shrimp and squid. Cut cleaned shrimp and squid into small pieces about 1/2 inch each.
2. Combine 2 oz. cooked de-veined shrimp, 2 ozs. cleaned cut squid, 1 cup celery chopped fine, 1 tbs. lime juice, 1 tsp. lemon or lime zest.
3. Refrigerate the ceviche seafood salad for 1-4 hours.
4. Serve in a small cup or on a bed of vegetables. Makes 1 portion. Each portion equals 4 ozs. protein, 1 cup vegetable.

• *2 ozs. de-veined cooked shrimp* • *2 ozs. cleaned cut pre-boiled squid* • *1 cup celery* • *1 tbs. lime or lemon juice* • *1 tsp. lime or lemon zest.*

Serving amount: 4 ozs. protein, non-aerosol oil mist

Chicken & Vegetables - Mixed Grille for Indoor or Outdoor Grill

1. Start cooking zucchini and green peppers first, as they take the longest to cook.
2. Remove from grill.
3. Then cook tomatoes and onions.
4. Remove from grill.
5. Then cook protein. 6. Weigh & measure for 16ozs vegetables and 4 ozs protein.

• *zuchini* • *green/red/yellow peppers*
• *onions tomatoes* • *5-6 ozs. protein (chicken, salmon, shrimp, catfish, tilapia, chilean sea bass, london broil, lamb, steak, chicken livers, chops, hamburger, turkey burger, salmon burger, hard tofu) before cooking*

Serving amount: 4 ozs. Protein, 1 1/2 cups vegetable

Chicken a la Lavender Cream

1. Cut chicken into bite-sized pieces.
2. Spray non-aerosol oil mist into a large deep frying pan and brown chicken lightly on all sides.
3. Reduce heat to medium and add garlic, herbs, and vinegar to deglaze the pan.
4. When vinegar has evaporated, add the soycream cheese, salt and pepper, and water or soymilk.
5. Stir until the soy cream cheese dissolves into a smooth sauce.
6. Reduce heat to very low and simmer for about 15 minutes or until sauce clings solidly to chicken. Makes 6 portions. Each portion equals 4 ozs. protein.

• *1 pound boneless chicken or 2 roasting hens or cornish hens, skin removed* • *non-aerosol oil mist*
• *2 cloves garlic,chopped* • *1 tsp. combination marjoram/thyme/summer savory/basil/rosemary/ fennel seeds* • *1 tsp. lavender flowers*
• *2 tbs. white vinegar* • *4 ozs. or ½ cup soy cream cheese* • *1 cup soy milk or water* • *salt and pepper.*

Serving protein: 1 oz. dairy/protein, 3 ozs. animal protein, non-aerosol oil mist

Protein - Animal & Soy

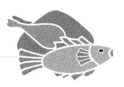

Chicken Alfredo

1. Place chicken in a single layer in a glassbaking dish and bake at 350 degrees for 30-40 minutes or until well-done but not dried out.
2. Remove chicken from pan, allow to cool,and cut into bite-sized pieces.
3. Drain off excess chicken fat but leave some in the pan.
4. Place pan over a burner on the stove and sauté the chopped garlic.
5. Add 1 cup water, bring to a boil, reduce heat, and simmer for 10 minutes, scraping up garlic from the bottom of the pan.
6. Add soy cream cheese and soy parmesan and cook, stirring, until well-blended.
7. Add salt and pepper to taste and return chicken to pan. Allow to heat through. Makes 6 portions. Each portion equals 4 ozs. protein.

- *1 pound boneless chicken, skin removed*
- *2 cloves garlic• 1/2 cup soy parmesan*
- *1/4 cup soy cream cheese • salt and pepper.*

Serving amount: 1 oz. dairy/protein, 3 ozs. animal protein, non-aerosol oil mist

Chicken Bog

1. Boil chicken with salt in 6 cups water until tender. (About 1 hour.)
2. Remove chicken, let cool and remove bones.
3. Chop meat in bite-sized pieces.
4. Skim off fat from juices.
5. Measure 3 1/2 cups of this broth into a 6-qt saucepan.
6. Add soy tofu nuggets, chicken pieces and smoked sausage, herb seasoning and poultry seasoning.
7. Cook these ingredients for 30 minutes.
8. Let come to a boil and turn to low, keeping covered the entire time. If mixture is too juicy, cook uncovered until desired consistency. If you use already-cut or boneless chicken, reduce the boiling time accordingly.

- *1 3 pound chicken • 1 tb salt • 1 cup soy tofu nuggets • 1/2 pound smoked sausage sliced*
- *1 tb onion powder • 2 tbs. mixed herbs*
- *1 tb. sage • 1 tbs. rosemary. Makes 10 portions. Each portion equals 4 ozs. protein*

Serving amount: 4 ozs. protein

Protein - Animal & Soy

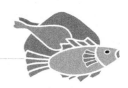

Chicken Breast, Legs or Thighs - Stewed or Roasted with Seasonings

1. Mix all spices together in small bowl.
2. Using a whole chicken fryer, carefullyseparate the skin from the meat and sprinklerub in between the skin and meat.
3. Gently rub the outer skin of the chickenwhere the spices were placed.
4. Refrigerate the chicken for 1 hour.
5. Roast in oven at 350 degrees until internaltemp is 160 degrees. If available, rotisseriechicken for 1 1/4 hours.
6. Measure 4 ounces and serve.

• 1 whole chicken fryer • 2 tsp.coriander, ground• 2 tsp. cumin, ground • 2 tsp. garlic powder• 2 tsp. marjoram, ground • 2 tsp.nutmeg,ground • 2 tsp.onion powder • 1 tsp. salt• 2 tsp. thyme, ground.

Serving amoung: 4 ozs. protein

Chicken Breasts Diane

1. Wash chicken breasts, pat dry, and sprinkle with salt and pepper.
2. Heat olive oil in a skillet and fry chicken breasts over high heat for 4 minutes on each side.
3. Transfer chicken to a warm serving platter, lower heat, and add the chives, lemon juice, parsley and mustard to the pan.
4. Cook, whisking constantly, for 15 seconds.
5. Add 2 tbs. water and stir until the sauce is smooth.
6. Return chicken to the pan and cook until just heated through.

• 2 large boneless chicken breast halves
• 2 tbs. olive oil • 1/2 tsp salt
• 1/2 tsp. black pepper • 3 tbs. chopped fresh parsley • 3 tbs. chopped fresh chives
• 2 tbs. mustard • 1 tb. lemon juice

Serving amount: 4 ozs. protein

Chicken Breasts, Sauteed

1. Spray skillet with zero-calorie butter spray.
2. Add soy sauce and garlic powder to skillet.
3. Add chicken breasts.
4. Cook until no longer pink.
5. Measure 4 ounces and serve.

• 4 boneless skinless chicken breasts • non-aerosol oil mist • 1 tsp. soy sauce or Bragg's Amino Acids (tastes like soy sauce only less sodium)
• 1/4 tsp. garlic powder

Serving amount: 4 ozs. protein

Protein - Animal & Soy

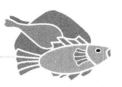

Chicken Chaat

1. Wash and cut the chicken into one inch pieces.
2. Spray pan with zero-calorie butter spray and heat.
3. Add garlic and salt.
4. Stri-fry the garlic and salt until it is light brown.
5. Add chicken pieces.
6. Stir-fry for 5-6 minutes, stirring constantly.
7. Add the masala powders.
8. Stir for another 3-4 minutes.
9. Check to see if the chicken is tender.
10. Remove from heat.
10. Weigh 4 ounces and serve. Option: Top chicken with 1 tsp. lemon juice.

• *1 boneless chicken breast* • *2-3 cloves garlic, peeled and chopped* • *zero-calorie butter spray*
• *1 1/2 tsp.dry coriander powder*
• *1/4 tsp. turmeric powder*
• *1/4- 1/2 tsp.red chili powder* • *salt*

Serving amount: 4 ozs. protein

Chicken Chimichurri

1. Put all ingredients for chimichurri sauce into blender or food processor and blend until smooth.
2. Put the sauce into a glass bowl or plastic food bag.
3. Add chicken; turn to coat well.
4. Marinate in the refrigerator at least 1 hour and up to 4 hours.
5. Prepare charcoal grill or heat broiler. While grill heats, soak wooden skewers in water at least 20 minutes so they don't burn.
6. Thread chicken onto skewers.
7. Grill, basting occasionally with the sauce, until chicken is no longer pink and edges are slightly golden, 10 to 15 minutes.
8. Serve immediately.

• *chimichurri sauce: 3 tbs. olive oil* • *1/2 cup fresh curly parsley chopped* • *1 tbs. fresh lemon juice* • *1 tsp. cracked black pepper* • *6 cloves garlic* • *1/2 teaspoon salt. poultry: 1 pound boneless skinless chicken breast cut into 1-inch wide strips*

Serving amount: 4 ozs. protein

Protein - Animal & Soy

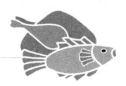

Chicken with Chipotle-Mustard

1. Whisk all ingredients except chicken together in an airtight container with a little water.
2. Marinate the chicken for at least one hour.
3. Grill over hot coals or bake in a 400 F oven until tender and just starting to brown. This has a lot of zip, but is not overwhelmingly hot.

- *2 cloves garlic pressed • 1 tsp. salt*
- *1 tsp. sweetener (optional) • 1 tb. apple cider vinegar • 1 tb. dijon mustard • 1 tb. chipotle purée • 1 tb. ground mustard • 2 tsp. dried thyme*
- *2 tsp. dried tarragon • 1 lb. boneless skinless chicken breasts or thighs*

Serving amount: 4 ozs. protein

Chicken - Jamacian Jerk Style

1. Place the hot pepper sauce in a shallow container.
2. Add chicken, one piece at a time, turning to coat.
3. Sprinkle salt, cinnamon and allspice over the chicken.
4. Place the chicken, skin side up, in a single layer in a large shallow baking dish lined with foil.
5. Bake at 400 degrees for 45 minutes or until the chicken is fork tender.

- *4 chicken quarters of the broiler/fryer type, skin removed • 1 tsp. salt • 1/2 tsp. cinnamon*
- *2 tbs. hot pepper sauce (e.g. tabasco)*
- *1/2 tsp. allspice*

Protein - Animal & Soy

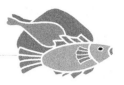

Chicken Liver Paté - Curried or Plain

1. Heat the oil in a deep, heavy frying pan over medium heat.
2. Sauté the chicken livers with the spices until they are barely pink inside, about 10 minutes.
3. Remove from heat and purée in a large food processor until smooth.
4. Pour paté into a container that will hold it comfortably and refrigerate until firm, at least 3 hours. Best the day after it is made, but actually just fine straight from the food processor.

•• *1 lb. chicken livers rinsed and trimmed • 1 tb. onion powder • 2 tsp. curry powder • 2 tsp. paprika, salt to taste • ½ tsp. black pepper • 2 tbs. extra virgin olive oil*

Serving amount: 4 ozs. protein

Chicken Mayan

1. Combine everything except the chicken and whisk until well mixed.
2. Add chicken and coat thoroughly.
3. Cover and chill 2-4 hours or overnight. Stir once in a while.
4. Grill over medium to hot oiled grill 5-7 min on each side until chicken is white in the center. Fairly hot and pleasantly tangy.
5. Reduce the quantity of chipotle purée if you need to.

• *3-4 garlic cloves, chopped*
• *2 tbs. chipotle purée*
• *2 tbs. fresh cilantro chopped*
• *2 tbs. achiote (annato) oil (or mix vegetable oil with 1 tsp. paprika)*
• *1 tb. balsamic vinegar*
• *2 kaffir lime leaves, boiled and soaked*
• *2 tsp. ground cumin*
• *2 tsp. dried oregano*
• *1/2 tsp. salt*
• *1/2 tsp. fresh ground pepper*

Protein - Animal & Soy

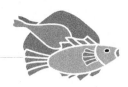

Chicken - Pollo Al Ajillo

1. Sprinkle the chicken with salt.
2. Heat the oil in a shallow flameproof casserole and brown the chicken on all sides over medium-high heat.
3. Add the chopped garlic, reduce heat to medium, and cook, stirring occasionally, for 30 minutes.
4. Stir in the minced garlic, parsley, and vinegar.
5. Cover and cook for 15 minutes more.

• *2 lbs. chicken meat, cut into small serving pieces* • *salt* • *3 tbs. olive oil* • *6 cloves garlic, coarsely chopped* • *1 clove garlic, pressed* • *1 tb. minced parsley* • *2 tbs. white vinegar*

Serving amount: 4 ozs. protein

Chicken - Sonoran

1. Poach chicken pieces until almost tender, about 15 minutes, in 1 quart of well-seasoned water, adding bay leaf, 2 garlic cloves, peppercorns, and salt.
2. Let chicken cool in broth.
3. Spray non-aerosol oil mist into a baking dish and lay the chicken on top of it.
4. Combine tomato paste, jalapeño powder, salt, black pepper, onion powder, and oregano with 2 cups reserved chicken stock in a saucepan.
5. Boil 5 minutes and add the remaining garlic.
6. Pour all of the sauce over the chicken, cover, and bake in 350 degree oven for 15 minutes, until bubbly. Makes 6 portions as chicken bones are removed. Each portion equals 4 ozs. protein, .50 oz. or 1/16 cup vegetable

---

• *2 lbs. chicken pieces, skin removed* • *1 quart water* • *1 bay leaf* • *2 cloves garlic, peeled and flattened, a few whole black peppercorns* • *1 tb. salt* • *1 tb. onion powder* • *non-aerosol oil mist* • *1/4 cup tomato paste* • *1 tsp. jalapeño powder* • *1/2 tsp. oregano* • *4 cloves garlic pressed.*

Serving amount: 4 ozs. protein, .50 or 1/16 cup vegetable

Protein - Animal & Soy

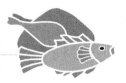

Chicken - Spicy Thai Style Ground with Basil

1. Heat oil in wok on high. Add chicken and stir fry 45 sec.
2. Add garlic and hot pepper flakes.
3. Cook until the chicken is no longer pink, about 2-3 minutes.
4. Add onion powder, lemon juice, soy sauce, and sweetener.
5. Stir-fry 30 seconds. 6. Add basil immediately before removing from heat and stir until it is just wilted

---

• *1 tb. vegetable oil* • *1 tb. hot oil* • *12 ozs. ground chicken, turkey, or beef* • *1 tb. onion powder*
• *1 tb. lemon juice* • *2 cloves garlic, minced*
• *1/2 tsp. red pepper flakes* • *2 tbs. soy sauce*
• *1 tsp. liquid sweetener* • *1/2 cup fresh basil leaves chopped*

Chicken - Sunset Barbecue

1. If you are using an oven broiler, heat oven (not broiler) to 450 degrees.
2. Rinse chicken and pat dry.
3. Set chicken on grill for 20 minutes, not directly over heat.
4. Cover the grill and open the vents o rplace chicken in a foil-lined pan and roas tfor 20 minutes.
5. While the chicken is pre-cooking, whisk the remaining ingredients together in a small bowl.
6. If you are using an oven broiler, remove chicken from oven, and pre-heat the broiler.
7. Brush half of this mixture on top of the chicken.
8. Return chicken to heat for 5 minutes.
9. Turn chicken and baste underside with the remaining sauce.
10. Cook until meat is no longer pink at the bone in the thickest part or about 5 minutes. The mustard coating should not be burnt. Makes 6-8 portions after chicken is off the bone. Each portion equals 4 ozs. protein.

• *2-3 pounds chicken pieces, skin removed* • *1 tsp. sweetener (optional)* • *2 tbs. dijon-style mustard* • *1 tsp. grated fresh ginger* • *1 clove garlic, pressed* • *salt and pepper.*

Serving amount: 4 ozs. protein

Protein - Animal & Soy

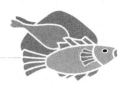

Chicken with 50 cloves of garlic

1. Place olive oil in a heavy pot which can be tightly covered.
2. Add 1/3 of garlic and 1/3 of all remaining ingredients, including chicken.
3. Add a second third of garlic and of the other ingredients.
4. Add remaining chicken and remaining ingredients.
5. Then cover pot tightly and place in a 375 F oven for about 1 hour and 15 minutes.
6. The chicken will not brown, but will be moist and succulent.
7. Purée the softened garlic cloves and sauce before serving.

• *3 tbs. olive oil* • *40-60 (that's right!) plump garlic cloves peeled* • *2 pounds boneless, skinless chicken thighs* • *1/2 cup chopped parsley*
• *1 tsp. dried tarragon* • *1 tb. salt*
• *1 tsp. white pepper* • *1/2 tsp. ground allspice*
• *1/4 tsp. cinnamon* • *3 tb white vinegar*

Serving amount: 4 ozs. Protein

Chicken - Yucatan Shredded

1. Place the peppercorns, oregano, and salt in a spice or coffee grinder and grind to a powder.
2. Combine this powder with the onion powder, the first two cloves garlic and the vinegar and make a paste.
3. Set aside.
4. Roast both heads of garlic in a 350° oven for 20 minutes and allow to cool. (Be sure they are truly cooked to liquid mushiness, or there will be a harsh taste to your chicken.)
5. Place the chicken in a stockpot with water to cover, dried habañero, salt, and oregano, and simmer until the chicken is tender, about 30 minutes.
6. Drain the chicken, reserving the broth, and transfer it to an oven-proof dish.
7. Add the peppercorn paste and bake uncovered at 350° until golden brown, about 30 minutes.
8. Peel the roasted garlic and combine it with the reserved chicken stock.
9. Add the chiles and simmer for 5 minutes.
10. Add the kaffir lime leaves, bring to a boil, and remove from heat immediately. When cool, purée in a blender.
11. Skin the chicken and shred the meat from the bones.
12. Add the purée to the chicken and mix well. 13. Heat through. This dish should be thick but not soupy.

• *10 peppercorns* • *1/4 tsp. ground oregano* • *1/2 tsp. salt* • *2 cloves garlic, pressed* • *1 tb. vinegar*
• *1 tb. onion powder* • *2 whole heads garlic* • *2 kaffir lime leaves soaked* • *3 lbs. chicken thighs*
• *1 tsp. salt* • *1/2 tsp. ground oregano 1 dried habañero chile*

Serving amount: 4 ozs. protein

Protein - Animal & Soy

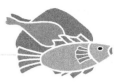

Clams, Steamed

1. Wash clams thoroughly, scrubbing under cold running water.
2. Place in large kettle or Dutch oven, on rack, so clams don't touch bottom.
3. Sprinkle with seasonings.
4. Add water, cover tightly, snf bring to a boiling point.
5. Steam just until shells open, about 5 minutes.
6. Discard any that do not open.
7. Remove clams from shells
8. Weigh 4 ozs.
9. Serve with allowable portion of butter.

- *3 pounds clams in shell • 1 1/2 cups water*
- *seafood seasoning • 1/4 tsp. thyme (optional)*
- *1-2 sprigs parsley, salt, pepper*
- *allowable portion of butter.*

Serving amount: 4 oz. protein

Clam & Cod Chowder - No Butter or Cream

1. Steam clams (as in recipe above) or use 4 ozs. diced clams. Save clam broth.
2. If using natural clam broth from steamed clams, filter broth in a coffee filter.
3. Put steamed clams or diced clams, fresh cod and other ingredients in a stock pot or sauce pan.
4. In a saute pan, use non-aerosol oil mist to saute 1 chopped onion or 1 cup leeks, 1 1/2 cups chopped celery, 2 cloves garlic, and

5. Add the chopped and browned garlic, bacon and onions to clams and cod.
6. Stir in 2 cups unsweetened soymilk.
7. Heat on medium and cook for 20-25 minute Do not boil or scald. Stir often.
Makes 4 portions. Each portion equals 1 prot (2 ozs. animal protein and 1/2 cup soy protein 1/2 cup vegetable

---

- *4 ozs. clams*
- *3 ozs. cod*
- *1 1/2 cup chopped celery*
- *1/2 cup chopped onion*
- *1 tbs. Old Bay Spice Blend*
- *2 cloves garlic*
- *1 oz. bacon*
- *2 cups unsweetened soymilk*

Serving amount: 1 protein, 1/2 cup vegetable

Protein - Animal & Soy

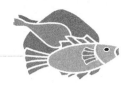

Eggs - Deviled

1. Hard boil the eggs. When slightly cool, cut the hardboiled eggs in half Scoop out the yolk and put in a small bowl.
2. Mix the yolk with the olive oil, the mustard and the Tabasco. When thoroughly mixed, spoon the egg mixture back into the egg-white halves.
3. Sprinkle with Paprika if you like.

- *2 hardboiled eggs • 2 tbs. olive oil*
- *1/4 - 1 tsp. dry mustard or wet mustard to taste*
- *1/2 - 1 tsp. tabasco sauce (what makes them a 'deviled' egg) (optional)*

Serving amount: 4 ozs. protein

Fish in Soy Ginger Sauce

1. Combine soy sauce and ginger to make ginger sauce. 2. Steam 4 ounces fish and top with sauce.

---

4 ozs. fish • soy sauce • freshly grated ginger

Serving amount: 4 ozs. protein

Fish with Seasonings - Bluefish, Lemon Sole, Flounder, Halibut, Orange Roughy, Red Snapper, Tuna - Grilled, Sauteed, Broiled, Baked

1. Buy fresh fish from a known fish vendor. Fish that has been frozen and thawed and fish that has been left for days in a grocery store may be bad and a waste of money.
2. Spray non-aerosol oil mist in a frying pan, fish poacher, or glass dish to be filled with water to poach, or to roast the fish in a roaster oven.
3. If sauteeing, sautee the fish on both sides for about 5 minutes on both sides.
4. If poaching fill the fish poacher or glass dish with about 1 inch of water. Place the fish in the poaching dish. Place the poacher either on the stove and boil the water with fish about 10 minutes. Or place the water-filled-poaching dish in a roaster oven.dish in an oven.
5. If roasting, place the fish in a dish sprayed with non-aerosol oil mist. Bake or roast the fish for about 15 minutes at 325 degrees. Use any seasoning blend to cover fish before or after cooking. Makes 1 portion.

- *4 ozs. bluefish, lemon sole, flounder, halibut, orange roughy, red snapper, scrod, tuna*

Serving amount: 4 ozs. protein

Protein - Animal & Soy

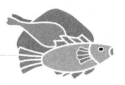

Lamb Chop or Roast with Garlic

1. Sprinkle lamb with fresh garlic minced or garlic powder, salt and pepper.
2. Cook until no longer pink or until done. Do not overcook.

• *4 ozs. lamb (chop or roast)* • *grated garlic*

Serving amount: 4 ozs. protein

Lamb Chops or Roast or Chunks - Broiled, Grilled as Kabobs or Roasted with Seasonings

1. Dice the meat into bite-sized cubes andsoak in warm water for 2-3 minutes.
2. Mix the paprika, ground coriander, salt, crushed garlic, onion powder, and cayenne pepper with the vinegar.
3. Drain the lamb and add to the marinade.
4. Marinate in the refrigerator for 6- 24 hours.
5. Heat the oil in a large heavy saucepan.
6. Add the black mustard seeds and stir a fewtimes.
7. Then add the ginger, cumin seeds, red chillies and turmeric powder.
8. Increase the heat and fry this masala for acouple of minutes.

9. Add the marinated lamb to the masala and mix well. At this point you have two options,either to cook the meat on the stove, in aslow cooker, or to bake it.
10. Stovetop cooking takes less time butrequires fairly constant stirring.
11. Leave meat in saucepan, reduce heat,cover, and stew over a low to medium flamefor about 45 minutes.
12. Add water if the sauce gets too dry andbegins to stick.
13. For baking, transfer meat and sauce to anovenproof casserole, cover it, and bake for 11/2 hours at 95 C .
14. Check occasionally, though you areunlikely to need to add any water to thesauce.
15. Finally, prepare and wash the fresh coriander in cold water. Only the leavesand the tender stems should be retained.
16. Chop coarsely and mix well just beforeserving. If you don't have any freshcoriander, use dried cilantro. Note: this works with beef, as well. The tougher the meat you start out with, the longer you should marinate it and the longer you should stew it.

• *4 ozs. lamb*
• *Spice Blend with ginger, cumin seeds, red chilies and turmeric powder for masala spice mix*

Serving amount: 4 ozs. protein

Protein - Animal & Soy

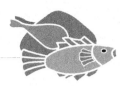

Lamb de Cordero

1. Cut the lamb into bite-sized chunks.
2. Trim off the excess fat and any gristle. Heat the oil in a wide saucepan.
3. Add the bay leaf and garlic and fry until the garlic is golden.
4. Discard the bay leaf. Take the pan off the heat and stir the paprika, onion powder, and chili powder into the oil, followed by the meat. Return to a gentle heat and pour in the vinegar.
5. Season and add the thyme.
6. Cover tightly and cook over a very low heat, stirring occasionally, until the meat is tender (10-15 minutes for leg meat, longer for stew meat). By this time the sauce should be thick and moist, not runny.

- *2 lbs. boned leg of lamb or lamb stew meat*
- *3 tbs. olive oil • 1 tb. onion powder*
- *4 - 5 cloves garlic sliced • 1 bay leaf*
- *1 tsp. spanish paprika (pimenton)*
- *pinch of chili powder • 3 tbs. balsamic vinegar*
- *salt and pepper • 1 sprig of fresh thyme*

Serving amount: 4 ozs. protein

Lamb - Ground with Persian Spices

1. Heat oil in a large skillet.
2. Add the ground lamb and cook until browned and crumbly.
3. Drain off fat, if necessary.
4. Add onion powder, allspice, curry powder, salt and pepper, and 2 Tb water to cooked meat.
5. Cook 3 minutes to blend flavors.
6. Add soy nuts, reduce heat and cover.
7. Simmer over low heat 15 minutes, stirring to prevent sticking.

- *2 tbs. almond oil • 1 tb. onion powder*
- *1 1/2 lbs ground lamb • 1/4 tsp. ground allspice • 1/4 tsp. madras curry powder*
- *salt and pepper to taste • 1/2 cup soy nuts*

Serving amount: 4 ozs. protein

Protein - Animal & Soy

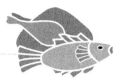

Lamb Stew In Tomato Sauce - Slow Cooker Method

1. In slow cooker place 1 1/2 cups crushedtomatos, 7 ozs fresh lamb cubes, 2 slicesbacon slicted thin and chopped, 1 tsp. nutmeg, 1 tsp. pepper.
2. Cook in slow cooker until the lamb istender.
3. May be cooked on low or high heat in slowcooker, depending on how fast you want it tocook. The tomato will thicken up. The lambwill develop a delicious taste.

- *1 1/2 cups crushed tomatos* • *7 ozs lamb cubes,*
- *1ozs uncooked no-sugar bacon* • *1 tsp. nutmeg,*
- *1 tsp.pepper.* • *makes 2 portions. each serving equals: 4ozs protein, 6 ozs or 3/4 cup vegetable*

Serving amount: 4 ozs. protein

Lamb Vindaloo

1. Sightly roast the cumin seed and coriander seed by frying with no oil for a minute or so, stirring constantly.
2. Grind these in a spice mill or coffee grinder and combine them into a paste with the other spices, the garlic, ginger, onion powder, tomato paste, and vinegar (not in the spice mill!).
3. Combine the lamb and the spice in a large bowl or container and mix well.
4. Refrigerate for 3-24 hours, mixing every few hours as convenient. (The marinating does add a lot of flavor and makes the meat much more tender, but if you are using a fairly tender cut of lamb, you can proceed directly from mixing to cooking.), When lamb has finished marinating, heat oil in a heavy-bottomed pan.
5. Add lamb and spice paste and simmer over low heat for half an hour.

- *2 lbs. cubed lamb* • *1 tb. coriander seed*
- *1/2 tbs. cumin seed* • *3 tbs. tomato paste*
- *14 cloves garlic pressed* • *6 bay leaves*
- *2-inch piece fresh ginger peeled and grated or finely chopped* • *1/2 tsp. ground black pepper*
- *1/2 tsp. cardamon seed* • *1/2 tsp. cinnamon*
- *1/2 tsp. cloves* • *1/2 tsp. cayenne*
- *1 tsp. ground mustard seed* • *1 tsp. turmeric*
- *1 tb. onion powder* • *3 tbs. cider vinegar*
- *3 tbs. olive oil*

Serving amount: 4 ozs. protein

Protein - Animal & Soy

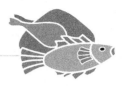

Mahi Mahi with Horseradish

1. Buy fresh fresh fish or only eat in a restaurant known to buy very fresh food and to have safe handling.
2. Wash hands before handling fish.
3. Take fish fillet and place in a frying pan with non-aerosol oil mist.
4. Cook 5 minutes on each side or until fish is very white and flaky.
5. Serve with wasabi (horseradish) or horserash. Makes 1 portion. Portion equals 4 ozs. protein served with salad.

- *4 ozs. mahi-mahi fillet • non-aerosol oil mist*
- *1 tb. wasabi or horseradish*

Serving amount: 4 ozs. protein, 12 ozs. vegetable

Meatballs with Lemongrass

1. Combine seasonings in a small bowl.
2. Place ground meat in a large bowl, pour seasonings over it, and combine thoroughly.
3. Cover and refrigerate for several hours or overnight.
4. Preheat oven to 350°.
5. Form marinated meat into 1-2 inch diameter meatballs and place on a foil-covered baking sheet.
6. Bake for approximately 30 minutes.

- *2 tbs. soy sauce • 1 tb. white vinegar*
- *2 1/2 tbs. fresh or 1 tb. dried lemon grass*
- *1 tb. peanut oil (optional) • 2 cloves garlic pressed or 1 tb. garlic powder • 1 tsp. red pepper flakes • 1/4 cup fresh or 1 tb. dried mint leaves*
- *1 tsp. liquid sweetener • 1 lb ground beef (or other ground meat)*

Serving amount: 4 ozs. protein

Protein - Animal & Soy

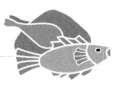

Meatballs Lucanian

1. Preheat oven to 350 °.
2. Combine ingredients thoroughly in a large mixing bowl.
3. Mold into small meatballs and place on foil- lined baking sheet.
4. Bake for about 30 minutes.

- *1/2 tsp. pepper • 1/2 tsp. cumin*
- *1 tsp. savory • 1 tb. parsley • pinch of rosemary*
- *1/4 tsp. ground cloves • 1 lb. ground meat*

Serving amount: 4 ozs. protein

Meatballs Moroccan

1. Mix meat with all seasonings and pound or knead vigorously until very smooth and pasty.
2. Shape small lumps of the mixture around skewers.
3. Grill, or bake on foil-covered tray, less the skewers.

- *2 lbs. finely ground beef • 2 tbs. onion powder*
- *3 tbs. parsley flakes • 1/2 tsp. marjoram • 1/4 tsp. ground cumin • 1/4 tsp. ground coriander*
- *1/2 tsp. harissa, salt and black pepper, 1/4 tsp. cayenne*

Serving amount: 4 ozs. protein

Meatballs - Moroccan Style

1. Mix meat with all seasonings and pound or knead vigorously until very smooth and pasty.
2. Shape small lumps of the mixture around skewers.
3. Grill, or bake on foil-covered tray, less the skewers.

- *2 lbs. finely ground beef*
- *2 tbs. onion powder*
- *3 tbs. parsley flakes • 1/2 tsp. marjoram*
- *1/4 tsp. ground cumin*
- *1/4 tsp. ground coriander*
- *1/2 tsp. harissa, salt and black pepper,*
- *1/4 tsp. cayenne*

Serving amount: 4 ozs. protein

Protein - Animal & Soy

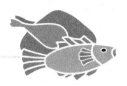

Meat - Spiced East Indian

1. After the meat has marinated, pour contents of the bowl into a wide 4-quart cooking pot.
2. Add the fennel and onion seeds. Bring to a boil.
3. Cover, lower heat, and simmer about 1 hour.
4. Lift off cover, raise heat, and boil rapidly until most of the liquid evaporates.
5. Now add the oil and keep stirring and frying over a medium flame. A thickish sauce should cling to the meat, which browns as the liquid cooks down.

• 2 1/2 lbs. cubed beef • 2 tbs. onion powder, a piece of fresh ginger, 2 inches long and 1 inch wide coarsely chopped • 6 cloves garlic pressed • 1 tb. ground coriander • 2 tsp. ground cumin • 1 tsp. ground turmeric • 1/8- 1/2 tsp. cayenne • 3 tbs. cider vinegar (optional) • 1 tsp. salt • 2 tsp. whole fennel seeds • 1 tsp. whole black onion seeds (kalonji) • 3 tbs. vegetable oil

Serving amount: 4 ozs. protein

Pork Chops or Roast - Broiled, Grilled as Kabobs or Roasted with Seasonings

1. Take small loin of pork or 2 pork chops.
2. Put in a pan.
3. Put pan in a 350 degree oven.
4. Roast about 30-45 minutes until no longer pink.
5. Pieces of pork loin may be cut and placed on skewers and grilled as kabobs. Makes 4 portions. Each portion equals 4 ozs. protein.

• 1 lb. pork loin • salt • 6 cloves garlic, coarsely chopped • 1 clove garlic, pressed • 1 tb. minced parsley • May be cooked and eaten plant with salt and pepper only.

Serving amount: 4 ozs. protein

Protein - Animal & Soy

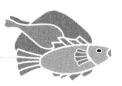

Pork Loin or Pork Chop Stuffed

1. Butterfly pork, starting at one long side and cutting horizontally to within 1 inch of opposite long side. Open as if it were a book.
2. Place a large sheet of plastic wrap over the veal and pound to 1/2-inch thickness, forming a rectangle approximately 10x12 inches.
3. Discard plastic and season pork with salt and pepper.
4. Combine soy cream cheese, chives, and roasted garlic in a bowl and beat until smooth.
5. Blanch the basil leaves in boiling water until just wilted, drain, and rinse with cold water.
6. Brush tomato paste along the center of the pork, forming a strip 2 inches wide.
8. Spoon soy cream cheese mixture on top of tomato paste in an even log. Arrange basil leaves in an overlapping layer on top. Fold one long side of pork over filling and roll tightly.
7. Cover ends of veal roil with heavy-duty aluminum foil to enclose filling completely.
12. Tie kitchen string around veal rolls every 1 1/2 inches to maintain neat log shape.
8. Wrap string lengthwise around veal roil to secure foil at ends, weaving string alternately under and over crosswise ties.
9. Cover and refrigerate until well chilled, at least 6 hours.
10. Preheat oven to 375° F.
11. Heat olive oil in a large heavy roasting pan over medium-high heat.
12. Season pork with salt and pepper, place in the pan, and brown on all sides, turning frequently, about 10 minutes.
13. Remove pan from heat and cool for 15 minutes. Drape bacon slices over pork, tucking the ends under the roast.
14. Roast pork in oven until a meat thermometer inserted into the center of the meat (not the filling) reads 140° F, about 45 minutes. Transfer to work surface and let stand 15 minutes.
15. To serve, remove bacon, string, and foil from pork roast. Cut roast crosswise into even slices.

- *1 center-cut veal or pork rib roast (rack of veal)*
- *about 4 1/2 lbs. boned and trimmed of all fat and outer membrane* • *salt and pepper*
- *1 container soy cream cheese* • *2 tbs. chives*
- *1 oz roasted garlic* • *16 large fresh basil leaves*
- *2 tbs. tomato paste* • *2 tbs. olive oil*
- *8 slices bacon*

Serving amount: 4 ozs. protein

Protein - Animal & Soy

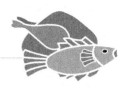

Salmon Loaf or Patties

1. Open and drain 16 or 12 oz. can of salmon.
2. Chop and measure onion and green pepper.
3. Mix all ingredients well and mash together.
4. Spray small loaf pan with non-aerosol oil mist.
5. Shapoe mixture in loaf pan into small loaf.
6. Bake loaf at 350 degrees for 20 minutes.
7. Be careful not to overcook.

Makes 3 or 4 portions, depending on size of can of salmon; 3 portions if using a 12 ozs. can, 4 portions if using a 16 ozs. can of salmon.

- *16 oz. can of Alaska salmon*
- *½ cup chopped onion*
- *½ cup chopped green pepper*
- *2 oz. oat bran*

Serving amount: 4 ozs. protein, ¼ cup vegetable, ½ oz. starch/grain

Salmon, Poached or Grilled with Cucumber, Spinach or Asparagus

1. Thinly slice raw cucumber to make ½ cup, or cook ½ cup spinach or asparagus.
2. Take ¼ red pepper or 1 tsp Tabasco sauce and mix with the vegetable you are using, Mix in the 1 tsp. lemon juice
3. Poach or grill 4 ozs. salmon
4. Cover the salmon with the thinly sliced raw cucumber, cooked spinach or asparagus for a lovely presentation and taste.

- *4 ozs. salmon*
- *½ cup thinly sliced raw cucumber, cooked spinach or cooked asparagus*
- *1 tsp. lemon juice*
- *¼ tsp. red pepper or 1 tsp. Tabasco sauce*

Serving amount: 4 ozs. protein, ½ cup vegetable

Protein - Animal & Soy

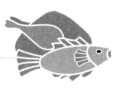

Sashimi

1. Buy fresh fresh fish or only eat in a restaurant known to buy very fresh food and to have safe handling.
2. Wash hands before handling fish.
3. Cut raw fish into small 1-2 inch pieces.
4. Refrigerate.
5. Take out of refrigerator 30 minutes only before serving. Makes 1 portion. Portion equals 4 ozs. protein served with salad.

• *4 ozs. sashimi (raw tuna, salmon, yellowtail)*
• *1 tb. ginger dressing • 1/2 cup boiled cold carrots • 1 cup salad with tomato and cucumber*
• *sashimi condiments: wasabi (horseradish mustard)*

Serving amount: 4 ozs. protein, 12 ozs. vegetable

Sausage & Cheese Quiche

1. Mix ingredients together well. 2. Microwave in a small bowl 1-2 minutes.

• *1 egg whipped • 1 oz. ground sausage or turkey sausage • 1 oz. soy cheese or regular cheese, grated or cubed • non-aerosol oil mist*

Serving amount: 4 ozs. protein

Sausage & Wild Mushrooms

1. Turn down to medium low and simmer until the juice is cooked down, stirring frequently(10-15 minutes.)

• *3 lbs fresh wild mushrooms thinly sliced*
• *1 lb hot italian sausage • 1 28 ozs. can whole tomatoes; 3 cloves garlic • 1/2 c olive oil*
• *1/4 - 1/2 tsp. crushed red pepper • salt and pepper to taste*

Serving amount: 4 ozs. protein

Sausage Eggplant Jumbalaya

1. Before dicing, slice and salt eggplant and let it "bleed" for about an hour and rinse.
2. Spray a skillet with PAM, add olive oil and heat.
3. Put the sausage around the outside of pan. In the middle, drop the eggplant and onion.
4. Cover and cook for about 30 minutes, stirring as needed.
5. Add the tomatoes and sprinkle on Greek Seasoning.
6. Cover and cook another 15 minutes or so.
7. Salt and pepper to taste. 8. Pan-fry.

• *1 1/2 cups diced eggplant • 1/2 cup diced onion • 1 cup diced tomato • 1 tsp. olive oil (optional) • 4 ozs. sweet italian sausage*
• *Greek seasoning*

Serving amount: 4 ozs. protein

Protein - Animal & Soy

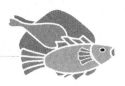

Scallops in Ginger

1. Thinly slice raw ginger root.
2. Spray a frying pan or wok with non-aerosol oil mist
3. Saute scallops and ginger for 4-6 minutes in sauté pan or wok.

- *4 ozs. bay or sea scallops*
- *1 tbs. thinly sliced fresh ginger root*
- *Non-aerosol oil mist*

Serving amount: 4 ozs. protein

Soynuts Roasted

1. Soak your beans covered in water for at least 12 hours or over n night.
2. Drain.
3. Spread them out on a cookie sheet in a single row, or as single as possible.
4. Spray with a little non-stick or use a spray of oil. I added same salt and garlic powder.
5. Cook at 325 for 1-3 hours stirring occasionally. They should get brown and crunchy. Or if you like them a little softer stop sooner. You can't taste for doneness. Squeeze a nut and see how it goes.

- *soy nuts*

Serving amount: 4 ozs. protein

Souvlakia

"For the vegetables, combine marinade ingredients with about 1 cup water in a large saucepan and bring to a boil.
1. Drop in mushrooms and stir to coat, about 1 minute.
2. Drop in onions and green pepper, ditto.
3. Remove pan from heat and let stand uncovered until cool.
4. Add tomatoes and stir thoroughly.
5. Transfer to a large container, cover, and marinate overnight in the refrigerator.
For the meat, combine marinade ingredients in a large container.
1. Add the meat and stir to coat thoroughly.
2. Marinate in the refrigerator overnight.
3. When the meat and vegetables have been thoroughly marinated, either thread them onto skewers and barbecue them or broil them in the oven."

- *meat: 2 lbs. lamb or beef cut into large chunks*
- *2 large yellow onions peeled and cut into quarters • 2 large green bell peppers cut into 1 1/2-inch chunks • 1 lb. fresh white mushrooms cleaned • 6 plum or cherry tomatoes • left whole, marinade (make 1 for meat, 1 for vegetables)*
- *3 tbs. good olive oil • 2 tbs. balsamic vinegar*
- *1 tb. lemon juice • 3 cloves garlic pressed*
- *2 bay leaves crumbled • 2 tbs. fresh or dried basil*
- *2 tbs. dried oregano • pinch thyme*
- *pinch crushed rosemary • salt and pepper to taste*

Serving amount: 4 ozs. protein

Protein - Animal & Soy

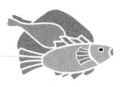

Tofu - Baked Ginger Shoyu Seasoned

1. Set the block of tofu on a cutting board with the longer end of the block facing you. Using a serrated knife, cut the tofu crosswise into nine slices, each a scant 1/2 inch thick. Cut each slice in half to create 2 squares. Set aside.

2. Place a rack in the center of the oven. Preheat the oven to 450 degrees. In a 10- or 12-inch skillet, combine the water, shoyu, ginger, garlic, star anise (if using), and red pepper flakes. Arrange the tofu squares in the marinade in one layer. Over high heat, bring to a boil. Cover, reduce the heat to medium-low, and simmer for 15 minutes.

3. Meanwhile, brush the sesame oil on the bottom of a large, shallow baking dish (about 7 by 11 inches). When the tofu squares are ready, carefully remove them one by one from the simmering marinade, brush off any bits of garlic or ginger, and set in the baking dish. Flip over each piece so that the second side gets a light coating of the oil. Sprinkle with 1 teaspoon of the sesame seeds. Bake uncovered until the top is a deep caramel-brown, 15 to 20 min¬utes. Flip over, sprinkle with the remaining sesame seeds, and bake until the second side is deeply browned, about 15 minutes more.

4. Remove the baking dish from the oven and set on a rack. The tofu will become firmer as it cools. When cool, refrigerate in a tightly sealed container until needed, up to 1 week.

• *1 pound extra-firm tofu, drained and pressed* • *l 1/4 cups water* • *1/4 cup shoyu or braggs amino acids that taste like soy sauce but have less sodium* • *1 tb. coarsely chopped fresh ginger* • *1 tb. coarsely chopped garlic* • *4 star anise, broken into petals (optional)* • *1/4 tsp. crushed red pepper flakes* • *1 1/2 tsp. toasted asian sesame oil* • *2 tsp. sesame seeds. Measure 4 ozs. for non-dairy protein.*

Serving amount: 4 ozs. protein

Protein - Animal & Soy

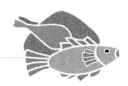

Tofu - Broiled Adobe Chipolte Barbecued

1. Chipotles in adobe is a thick paste of chipotles, vinegar, onions, garlic, and spices. Look for it in Hispanic groceries and gourmet shops. Chipotle chilies are dried jalapenos that impart a hot, smoky flavor. They may be purchased from gourmet shops either whole or ground. To grind your own, stem and seed the chili, snip it into bits, and grind the bits to a powder in a spice grinder.
2. Wrap the tofu in several layers of a clean, absorbent kitchen towel and set a 1-pound bag of dried beans on top. Set the tofu aside until you are ready to slice it.
3. Line a broiling pan or baking sheet with aluminum foil. Set aside. Place the oven rack about 5 inches from the broiling element, and turn on the broiler.
4. In a pie plate or large, shallow bowl, prepare the barbecue sauce by blending together the remaining ingredients.
5. Unwrap the tofu and Set the block on a cutting board with the longer side facing you. Cut the block crosswise into 9 slices, each slightly less than 1/2 inch thick. Dip the slices into the sauce to coat both sides heavily. Arrange the slices on the broiling pan as you work. (Reserve any remaining sauce.)
6. Broil the tofu until flecked with dark brown spots, 4 to 6 minutes. (If your broiler cooks unevenly, rotate the broiling pan halfway through.) Turn the tofu over with a spatula and slather any remaining sauce on the second side with a pastry brush or knife. Broil until deeply browned on the second side, 4 to 6 more minutes. Serve with the darker side up.

- *1 pound block extra-firm tofu, drained*
- *2 generous tbs. dijon mustard*
- *2 generous tbs. ketchup*
- *1 1/2 to 2 tbs. shoyu (depending upon desired saltiness)* • *1 large clove garlic, peeled and pushed through a press* • *2 tsp. blackstrap molasses*
- *2 tsp. toasted asian sesame oil* • *1 to 2 tsp. chipotle in adobo or 1/8 to 1/4 tsp. ground chipotle chili (see note) or cayenne pepper freshly ground black pepper, to taste*

Serving amount: 4 ozs. protein

Protein - Animal & Soy

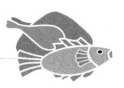

Tofu Curried With Spinach And Tomatoes

1. Set the block of defrosted tofu or fresh tofu between 2 plates and, pressing the plates firmly together, tip them over the sink as the tofu releases excess water. Release the pressure slightly, then press the plates firmly together again 4 or 5 more times, or until no more water is expressed. With a serrated knife, slice the tofu into 1-inch cubes. Set aside.

2. Put non-aerosol oil mist in a large, heavy saucepan or wok over medium-high heat. Saute the onions, stirring frequently, until lightly browned, about 3 minutes. Add the water and blend in the curry paste and no alcohol coconut flavoring. Stir in the reserved tofu, taking care to coat the tofu thoroughly with the curry sauce. Stir in the tomatoes.

3. Cover and cook over medium heat, stirring occasionally, until the tomatoes are soft, about 5 minutes. If the mixture seems quite dry, stir in 1/4 cup water at this point. Add the spinach. If your pot isn't big enough, you may need to add half, cover, and let it wilt before adding the remainder. Cover and continue cooking until the spinach is tender, 2 to 3 minutes. Add salt and the cilantro, if you like these flavors. Makes 4 portions. Each portion equals 4 ozs. protein, 12 ozs. or 1 1/2 cups vegetables, non-aerosol oil mist

• *1 lb. block extra-firm or firm tofu, frozen, defrosted, and drained or fresh • non-aerosol oil mist • 4 ozs. or l/2 cup coarsely chopped onions • 1 cup water • 1/4 cup mild curry paste • 4 ozs. or 4 large plum tomatoes, cored and cut int eighths • 16 ozs. or 1 pound spinach, trimmed, coarsely chopped, and thoroughly washed • salt, taste • 1/3 to 1/2 cup chopped cilantro (option*

Serving amount: 4 ozs. protein, 12 ozs. or 1/2 cups vegetable, non-aerosol oil mist

Protein - Animal & Soy

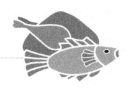

Tofu - Sauteed, Plain or Roasted with Seasonings

1. Set the block of defrosted tofu or fresh tofu between 2 plates and, pressing the plates firmly together, tip them over the sink as the tofu releases excess water. Release the pressure slightly, then press the plates firmly together again 4 or 5 more times, or until no more water is expressed. With a serrated knife, slice the tofu into 1-inch cubes. Set aside.
2. Put non-aerosol oil mist in a large, heavy saucepan or wok over medium-high heat.
3. Cover and cook over medium heat, stirring occasionally about 5 minutes. If the mixture seems quite dry, stir in 1/4 cup water at this point.
4. If roasting, place in a pan and place pan in roaster oven and roast at 325 degrees for about 15-20 minutes.
5. Add seasoning blends, if you like these flavors. Makes 4 portions. Each portion equals 4 ozs. protein, non-aerosol oil mist

---

• *1 lb. block extra-firm or firm tofu, frozen, defrosted, and drained or fresh* • *non-aerosol oil mist* • *salt, to taste*

Serving amount: 4 ozs. protein

Tuna Salad

1. Flake the tuna.
2. Combine with celery and onion.
3. Bind with allowable portion of mayonnaise.
4. Serve on greens.

• *1/2 cup white-meat tuna* • *1 cup finely cut celery* • *3/4 cup greens* • *1/4 cup finely chopped onion* • *1/2 tsp. salt* • *1/2 tsp. pepper* • *mayonnaise*

Serving amount: 4 ozs. protein

Turkey Burgers With Barbeque Sauce

1. Add all ingredients in a bowl.
2. Mix well.
3. Use generous helpings of spices andbarbecue sauce.
4. Either on a grill or in a frying panform into burgers and cook as you wouldhamburger.
5. Cook until done.

• *1 package ground turkey* • *onion powder* • *garlic powder* • *salt* • *pepper* • *use Texas Best "original recipe" bbq sauce caution: all other varieties of texas best are not abstinent.orbarbeque spice blend. (see barbeque blend inspice blend recipes).*

Serving amount: 4 ozs. protein

Protein - Animal & Soy

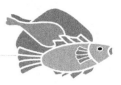

Turkey Breast Legs or Thighs - Poached or Roasted with Seasonings

1. Take turkey breast, drumsticks or thighs or whole turkey and wash under cold water.
2. If poaching or stewing fill the clow cooker or pot to be used for boiling with enough water to cover the turkey pieces. Place the pot on the stove and boil the water with the turkey or cook the turkey in the slow cooker on low or high. The slow cooker will make the turkey very cooked and moist. It will be easy to remove the turkey from the bones. Cool the turkey first in order to handle it easily and remove it from the bones easily. You may then make turkey soup, turkey salad, turkey with brown rice or freeze the turkey for future use in freezer bags.
3. If roasting, place the turkey in a pan for the oven or roaster oven. Bake or roast the turkey 325 degrees about 12 minutes per pound. Use any seasoning blend to cover turkey before or after cooking.

• *1-2 lbs. turkey breast, thighs or drumsticks or 10-20 lbs whole turkey* • *Seasoning blend (see Seasoning Blend Recipes)*

Serving amount: 4 ozs. protein

Starch/Grains & Beans/Legumes

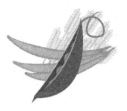

Bean Salad - Cold or Hot

1. Mix all ingredients together and chill.
2. Serve Cold or Heat 1 minute in Microwave.

• 1/4 cup chopped onion • 1/4 cup chopped pepper • 1/4 cup chopped parsley or 2 tbs. parsley flakes • 1/3 cup black beans cooked • 1/3 cup pink beans cooked • 1/3 cup red beans cooked or any 1 cup of a single type bean • 1/4 cup tomato chopped • 1 tsp. rosemary • 1 tsp. cilantro • 1 tsp. oil and vinegar dressing or oil and lemon

Serving amount: 1 cup cooked starch/grain/ beans/legumes, 3/4 cup vegetables, 1 tsp. oil

Brown Rice Custard - Brown Rice Pudding III

1. Mix egg with milk, rice, cinnamon and nutmeg.
2. Pour mixture into the small glass baking dish or loaf pan.
3. Place the glass fish or loaf pan in a shallow cooking dish filled with 1/2 inch water.
4. Pre-heat oven to 325 degrees.
6. Oven Bake - 325 degrees - estimated cooking time 25 minutes. Microwave - on High - estimated cooking time 6 minutes, or until liquid is absorbed.

• 1/2 cup cooked brown rice • 1 egg • 1 cup milk
• 1/4 tsp. cinnamon • 1/4 tsp. nutmeg
• sweetener (optional)

Serving amount: 1 protein, 1 dairy, 1/2 cup cooked starch/grain

Brown Rice - Cottage Cheese Rice Pudding IV

1. Mix ingredients.
2. Cook in microwave for 1-2 minutes.

• 1/2 cup cottage cheese • 2 tbs. water
• 1 cup cooked brown rice • 1/2 tsp. cinnamon

Serving: 1 protein or dairy, 1 cup cooked starch/grain

Brown Rice Pudding V - Tofu & Brown Rice

1. Blend tofu until smooth. Add brown rice.
2. Cook and stir over medium heat until the mixture thickens. Stir and watch so it does not burn.
3. To Bake: Pour into a small casserole dish.
4. Set casserole or glass dish into another pie plate of water so the water touches the sides of the casserole dish.
5. Bake for 15-20 minutes until semi-firm.
6. Cool. Serve.

• 4 ozs. silken tofu • 1 cup cooked brown rice
• 1/4 tsp. nutmeg

Serving amount: 1 protein or dairy-free substitute, 1 cup cooked starch/grain

Starch/Grains & Beans/Legumes

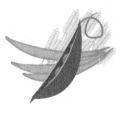

Cabbage Rolls with Brown Rice & Spiced Meat - Slow Cooker Method

1. Mix meat, 1/2 cup cooked brown rice and onions.
2. Peel cabbage leaves from whole cabbage. Peel so that cabbage leave are as whole as possible and as large as possible.
3. Measure cabbage leaves so that they equal 8 ozs or 1 cup cooked vegetable.
3. Place small amount of meat-rice mixture in center of one cabbbage leaf.
4. Roll cabbage leav, from the ends in first. It is alright if the leaf is somewhat loose. You may leave it loose.
5. Roll all the cabbage leaves with the meat mixture.
6. Drop the cabbage rolls into the 1 cup tomato sauce with 1 cup water in a slow cooker.
7. Cook in the slow cooker 1 hour on high or 2 hours on low.

• *5-1/2 ozs. chopped meat, turkey or beef (This may be Italian sausage taken out of the casement. You may add spices to the meat, including anise, parsley, sage, rosemary or any other spices you want)* • *1 cup tomato juice or 1 cup green pepper chopped fine* • *1 cup cooked brown rice (reserve 1/2 cup)* • *1 cup water* • *1/4 cup onion chopped* • *1 tsp. parsley* • *4-5 boiled cabbage leaves*

Serving amount: 1 protein, starch/grain, 2 vegetable

Chicken Or Turkey Soup with Brown Rice with Vegetables - Slow Cooker or Stove Method

1. Open large cans of crushed or stewed tomatoes. Chop carrots. Open frozen green beans and measure 1 cup. Place crushed tomatoes, turkey or chicken, 1 cup brown rice, carrots and green beans, spices in a slow cooker or large saucepan.
2. Cook stew on slow simmer for 2 hours.

• *1 1/2 cups crushed or stewed tomatoes (1 large can)* • *1 cup water* • *1 cup cooked or uncooked chopped green beans* • *1 cup carrots cut into small pieces* • *4 ozs chopped turkey or chicken* • *1 cup cooked brown rice* • *Herbes de Provence spice blend (see Spice Blend Recipes). Makes 2 portions. Each portion equals: 2 ozs protein (if prepared with turkey or chicken), 1/2 cup starch/grain, 1/2 cup starchy vegetable, 1 1/2 cups vegetable*

Serving amount: 2 ozs. protein, 1/2 cup starch/grain, 1/2 cup starchy vegetable, 12 ozs. or 1 1/2 cups cooked vegetable

Starch/Grains & Beans/Legumes

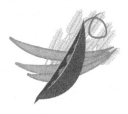

Chick Pea - Kidney Bean Herbes de Provence Salad - Hot or Cold

1. Stir-fry or saute onions and peppers until tender.
2. Mix cooked lentils with vegetables.
3. Heat for 15 minutes in microwave or on stove or in slow cooker (where you may cook the lentils).

Dried beans and lentils are extremely versatile. A staple of many a global cuisine, they can be made into wonderful soups, infused with herbs and vegetables. They can be used in salads sprinkled with lime juice. Beans also can be pureed and served as a dip or spread.

- *1 cup kidney beans*
- *1 cup chick peas • 1/2 cup chopped parsley*
- *dressing of choice*
- *Herbes de Provence (see Spice Blend Recipes). Makes 2 portions. Each portion equals 1 cup starch/grain/beans-legumes, 2 ozs. or 1/4 cup vegetable*

Serving amount: 1 cup starch/grain, 1/4 cup vegetable

Chick Peas with Lemon

1. Open can of chick peas.
2. Measure 1/2 cup per serving.
3. Add dill, chopped onions, lemon juice and oil. Toss. Measure serving and serve.

---

1 cup cooked chick peas ~ 1/4 c onions chopped ~ 1 tsp. dill weed or seed or 2 tbs. fresh dill ~ 1 1/2 tsp. olive oil ~ 1 tbs. lemon juice ~ 1/4 tsp. lemon peel

Serving amount: 1 cup cooked starch/grain/beans/legumes , 1 tsp. oil

Chili I - Pinto Bean - Kidney Bean Chili

1. Mix all ingredients in a saucepan.
2. Heat on slow simmer for 30 minutes. If chili gets too dry, add water.
3. Measure 1 cup and store leftovers for up to 3 days. Double recipe as needed for more servings to freeze or share.

- *1/2 cup cooked pinto beans • 1/2 cup cooked kidney beans • 1 minced garlic clove*
- *1/2 tbs. dried cilantro • Sonora spice blend (see Spice Blend Recipes)*

Serving amount: 1 cup cooked starch/grain

Starch/Grains & Beans/Legumes

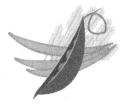

Chili II - Bean & Tofu Vegetarian Chili

1. Mix all ingredients in a saucepan.
2. Heat on slow simmer for 30 minutes. If chili gets too dry, add water.
3. Measure 1 cup and store leftovers for up to 3 days. Double recipe as needed for more servings to freeze or share.

• *1/2 cup cooked red beans* • *1/2 cup cooked black or kidney or pinto beans* • *1 minced garlic clove* • *4 ozs. tofu* • *1 cup red or green bell pepper* • *1/2 tbs. dried cilantro* • *Sonora spice blend (see Spice Blend Recipes)*

Serving amount: 4 ozs. protein, 1 cup vegetable, 1 cup cooked starch/grain

Chili III - Bean & Ground Beef Chili

1. Mix all ingredients in a saucepan.
2. Heat on slow simmer for 30 minutes. If chili gets too dry, add water.
3. Or. put slow cooker on low. Cook 2 hours. Or put slow cooker on high. Cook 1 hour. If chili gets too dry, add water.

• *1/2 cup cooked red beans* • *1/2 cup cooked black or kidney or pinto beans* • *1 minced garlic clove* • *4 ozs. ground beef* • *1 cup red or green bell pepper   1/2 tbs. dried cilantro* • *Sonora spice blend (see Spice Blend Recipes)*

Serving amount: 4 ozs. protein, 1 cup vegetable, 1 cup cooked starch/grain

Falafel I

1. Mash all ingredients together or pulse ingredients briefly in a blender or with a hand mixer.
2. Form mixture into small balls around 1-2 inches.
3. Heat oven to 325 degrees.
4. Saute falafel for 4-6 minutes, turning to brown each side, in a saute pan sprayed with non-aerosol oil mist.
5. Place balls on a baking sheet and bake for 15 minutes for a dryer cooked falafel.
6. Drain falafel on paper towels.

• *1/4 cup cooked brown rice*
• *3/4 cup cooked chick peas*
• *1/2 tsp. coriander*
• *1/2 tsp cumin*
• *1/4 tsp. black pepper*
• *1/2 tsp. parsley or cilantro*

Serving amount: 1 cup cooked starch/grain

Starch/Grains & Beans/Legumes

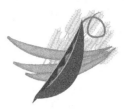

Falafel II
With Oat Bran

1. In a large bowl mash chickpeas until
thick and pasty; don't use a blender,
as the consistency will be too thin.
2. In a blender, process onion,
parsley and garlic until smooth.
Stir into mashed chickpeas.
3. In a small bowl combine egg, cumin,
coriander, salt, pepper, cayenne,
lemon juice and baking powder.
4. Stir into chickpea mixture.
Slowly add oat bran until mixture
is not sticky but will hold together.
5. Form 8 balls and then flatten into patties.
6. Spray skillet with non-aerosol oil mist.
Heat skillet over medium-high heat. Fry
patties in oil mist until brown on both sides.
7. Makes 3 portions. Each portion equals
1/3 protein, ½ cup vegetable and 1 cup
cooked starch/grain

• 1 (15 ounce) can chickpeas (garbanzo beans),
drained (2 cups) • 1 onion, chopped
• 1/2 cup fresh parsley • 2 cloves garlic, chopped
• 2 eggs • 2 tsp.ground cumin
• 1 tsp. ground coriander • 1 tsp. salt
• 1 dash pepper • 1 pinch cayenne pepper
• 1 teaspoon lemon juice • 1 tsp. baking powder
• 1/2 cup dry oat bran • Non-aerosol oil mist

Serving amount: ½ protein, ½ cup vegetable,
1 cup cooked starch/grain

Green Pepper Stuffed with
Ground Beef or Sausage Pieces
or Tofu & Brown Rice   -
Slow Cooker Method or Baked

1. Core a green peppers. Remove
seeds and leave bottom of each
pepper intact. 2. Measure 4 ozs. of
ground beef, sausage pieces or tofu
3. Mix protein with 1 cup cooked
brown rice. 4. Fill the green peppers
with the protein-brown rice mixture.
5. Pour 1 cup crushed tomatos over
the green peppers, either in the glass
baking dish if baking, or in the slow
cooker, if using the slow cooker method.
6.. Bake at 325 or 350 degrees. Or put the
green peppers in the slow cooker and cook
in the slow cooker - on Low 2 hour, on High
1-2 hours. Makes 2 portions. Each portion
equals 1/2 cup cooked brown rice and 8 ozs.
cooked vegetable

• 2 raw large green peppers (4 ozs. each)
• 4 ozs. ground beef, sausage pieces or tofu
• 1 cup chopped stewed tomatoes
• 1 cup cooked brown rice

Serving amount: 1/2 cup starch/grain, 8 ozs.
or 1 cup vegetable, 2 ozs. or 1/2 protein

Starch/Grains & Beans/Legumes

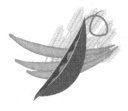

Hummus from Garbanzo Beans - Chick Peas

1. Pulse ingredients in a blender or food processor until mixture is smooth. Add a small amount of water to help blending if needed. Remove mixture from the blender.
3. Store in an airtight container for up to 4 days. May be served with raw vegetables.

• *1 cup cooked garbanzo beans* • *1 tbs. lemon juice*
• *1 tsp. sesame oil* • *1 tsp. minced garlic*
• *1 tsp. fresh chopped parsley* • *1/4 tsp. cumin or 1/4 tsp. red pepper flakes* • *Mideast Seasoning (see Mideast Price Blend). Makes 1 portion.*

Serving amount: 1 cup cooked starch/grain, 1 tsp. oil

Kasha and Onions

1. Saute onions in non-aerosol cooking spray.
2. Cook kasha (buckwheat groats).
Buckwheat is a different grain and not wheat.
3. Mix onions, kasha, oil and pepper.
4. Heat for 3 minutes.
5. Steam in microwave with 3 tbs water for reheating. Makes 2 portions. Each portion equals 1/2 cup cooked kasha and 1/4 cup vegetable

---

• *1 cup cooked kasha* • *1/2 cup chopped onions*
• *1 tsp. pepper* • *1/8 tsp. pepper*

g amount: 1/2 cup starch/grain, 2 ozs.
cup vegetable

Lentils Italian Style

1. Soak lentils for 2-3 hours in water.
2. Rinse and discard discolored lentils and stones.
3. Spray sautee pan with non-aerosol non-fat cooking spray.
4. Saute onions and garlic.
5. Cook lentils after soaking in 2 cups. water for only 25 minutes on low.
6. Drain lentils.
7. Place 1 cup lentils in pot.
8. Add remaining ingredients to lentils.
9. Simmer on low for 10 minutes. Water can be added if mixture gets dry. Lentils can be prepared Plain without added ingredients. They can be stored in airtight containers for up to 4 days. Makes 1 portion. Equals 1 cup cooked starch/grain/beans-legumes. Add Sonora Spice Blend, Moroccan Spice Blend or Italian Spice Blend (see Spice Blend Recipes)

• *1/2 cup dry lentils* • *1/2 cup cooked minced onion* • *2 minced garlic cloves* • *1/2 cup tomato sauce* • *1/2 cup chopped tomato* • *1 tsp. chopped parsley* • *1/2 tsp. Italian seasoning* • *1 cup vegetable broth. Sonora Spice Blend or Moroccan Spice Blend or Italian Spice Blend (see Spice Blend Recipes)*

Serving amount: 1 cup cooked starch/grain, 12 ozs. or 1 1/2 cup vegetable

Starch/Grains & Beans/Legumes

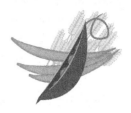

Lentils with Onions & Tomato with Green Pepper

1. Stir-fry or saute onions and peppers until tender. Mix cooked lentils with vegetables.
2. Heat for 15 minutes in microwave or on stove or in slow cooker (where you may cook the lentils). Measure 4 ozs. or 1/2 cup

---

- *1 cup cooked lentils • 1/4 tsp. oregano*
- *1 cup chopped stewed tomatoes*
- *1/4 tsp. celery seed • 1 cup chopped onions*
- *1/2 cup chopped pepper*

Serving amount: 1/2 cup cooked starch/ starch vegetable

Lentil & Brown Rice Lemon Soup

1. In a Dutch oven or heavy stock pot, heat the oil over medium heat. Add the onion and sausage, and cook, stirring frequently, until the sausage is lightly browned. Stir in the garlic, and cook for an additional 1 minute.
2. Add the lentils and brown rice to the pot along with the stock. Bring to the boil, then reduce heat to simmer. Cover the pot and cook for 1 hour, until the rice is tender.
3. Uncover, and stir in soy sauce, lemon rind, and black pepper. If the soup is too thick, add water, one cup at a time, to achieve the consistency you prefer. Taste, and adjust seasoning if necessary with salt
4. Serve hot, or allow to cool completely and freeze for up to six months. When you are ready to reheat, add water or more stock, as the lentils and rice will absorb every bit of liquid you give them. Makes 3 portions. Each portion equals 1 cup cooked starch/grain.

- *1 medium onion, diced*
- *1 large clove garlic, thinly sliced*
- *4 ozs. or 1/2 cup uncooked lentils*
- *2 ozs. or 1/4 cup uncooked brown rice*
- *9 cups stock (chicken or vegetable stock or water)*
- *1 tbs. soy sauce*
- *1-1/2 tbs. minced lemon rind*
- *dash black pepper • dash salt or more to taste*

Serving amount: 1 cup cooked starch/grain

Starch/Grains & Beans/Legumes

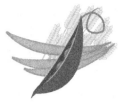

Mushroom Brown Rice & Miso Soup - Cremini, Shitake or Portobello Mushrooms

1. Break off the shiitake (or other) mushroom stems (or pry them out with a sharp paring knife). Discard the stems or reserve them for stock. Break or chop the shiitake caps into tiny bits. Quickly rinse and drain. Set aside.
2. In a large, heavy soup pot, heat the oil over high heat. Saute the garlic for 1 minute, stirring frequently. Add the thyme and continue cooking over high heat until about half evaporates.
3. Add the vegetable stock, reserved shiitakes, and brown rice, and bring to a boil. Reduce the heat to low, cover, and cook at a gentle boil until the barley is tender, 30 to 45 minutes.
4. Pour the hot water into a large glass measuring cup and dissolve 3 tablespoons of the miso in it by mashing the paste against the sides of the cup and stirring vigorously with a whisk or fork.
5. Turn off the heat and stir the miso broth into the soup. Taste and add the additional miso as needed for flavor, first dissolving the miso in a small amount of the soup's broth. Add salt, if needed. Ladle into bowls, garnish with the parsley, and serve immediately.

- *2 oz. dried shiitake mushrooms or 4 ozs. cremini or portobello mushrooms*
- *1 tsp. olive oil*
- *1 tsp. minced garlic*
- *1/2 tsp. dried thyme or marjoram leaves*
- *6 cups vegetable stock*
- *1 cup cooked brown rice* • *1/2 cup hot water*
- *3 to 4 tbs. sweet white miso*
- *3 tbs. minced parsley, for garnish*

Serving amount: 1 cup cooked starch/grain, 1 tsp. oil, 1/2 cup vegetable

Potato or Sweet Potato or Yam Baked, Roasted, Steamed or Microwaved

1. Choose a small potato or yam. Or cut a larger one in half. Take a fork and poke a few holes in the side of the potato to ease cooking and allow steam to escape.
2. Bake or Roast at 325 or 350 degrees for baked or roasted. Or microwave for 8 minutes on power 8. Makes 1 portion. Measure 4 ozs.

- *4 ozs. potato, sweet potato or yam.*

Serving amount: 1/2 cup cooked starch/ starch vegetable

Starch/Grains & Beans/Legumes

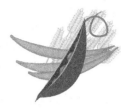

Quinoa I - Tabouli Style - Salad-Side

1. In a saucepan bring water to a boil. Add quinoa and a pinch of salt. Reduce heat to low, cover and simmer for 15 minutes. Allow to cool to room temperature; fluff with a fork.
2. Meanwhile, in a large bowl, combine sea salt, lemon juice, tomato, cucumber, and parsley. 3. Stir in cooled quinoa. Makes 2 portions. Each portion equals 1/2 cup cooked starch/grain and 1 cup vegetable

---

- *2 cups water • 1/2 cup uncooked quinoa*
- *1/2 tsp. sea salt • 1/4 cup lemon juice*
- *1/2 cup fresh tomato, diced finely*
- *1/2 cup cucumber, diced finely*
- *1 cup fresh parsley, chopped finely*

Serving amount: 1/2 cup cooked starch/grain, 1 cup vegetable

Quinoa II - Spicy Style

1. In a saucepan, combine the quinoa, water and salt. Bring to a boil, then reduce heat to medium and cook until quinoa is tender and water has been absorbed, about 10 minutes. Cool slightly, then fluff with a fork.
2. Transfer the quinoa to a serving bowl and stir in the lemon juice, celery, onion, cayenne pepper, cumin and parsley.
3. Adjust salt and pepper before serving. Makes 2 portions. Each portion equals 1/2 cup starch/grain and 1 cup vegetable.

- *1/2 cup uncooked quinoa*
- *2 cups water*
- *sea salt to taste*
- *1/4 cup fresh lemon juice*
- *3/4 cup fresh celery, chopped finely*
- *1/4 cup red onion, chopped finely*
- *1/4 tsp. cayenne pepper*
- *1/2 tsp. ground cumin*
- *1 cup fresh parsley, chopped inely*

Serving amount: 1/2 cup cooked starch/grain, 1 cup vegetable

Starch/Grains & Beans/Legumes

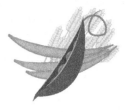

Red or Black Beans & Collard Greens

1. To prepare red or black beans, soak beans overnight to reduce cooking time.
2. Cook with water in a ratio of 3 to 1 - water to beans. Cook on medium heat or in slow cooker for about 2 hours, careful not to burn beans and that the water is absorbed and does not evaporate.
3. Wash fresh collard greens at least 3 times, carefully rinsing all leaves.
4. Cut end stems from collard greens. Either dice ends into small pieces, if you choose to eat them, or discard ends.
5. Boil collard greens in water until tender. Take kitchen shears and cut up large leaves into smaller bite-size amounts.
6. Serve the collard greens with the red or black beans. Makes 1 portion. Portion equals 1 cup cooked beans and 12 ozs. collard greens.

• *1/2 cup uncooked pinto beans, red beans or black beans*
• *water to soak beans overnight*
• *3 cups water to cook beans*
• *12 ozs. fresh collard greens*
• *1/2 tsp. cumin • 1 tbs. cooked minced onions*
• *Sonora Seasoning (see Sonora Spice Blend Recipe) for red or black beans.*

Serving amount: 1 cup cooked starch/grain/beans-legumes, 1 1/2 cup or 12 ozs. vegetable

Refried Beans

1. Pulse ingredients in a blender or food processor until mixture is smooth. Add a small amount of water to help blending if needed.
2. Remove mixture from the blender.
3. Store in an airtight container for up to 4 days.
4. May be heated. Makes 1 portion. Equals 1 cup cooked starch/grains/beans-legumes. May be divided into two portions of 1/2 cup cooked starch/grains/beans-legumes.

• *1 cup cooked pinto beans red beans or black beans • 1/2 tsp. cumin • 1 tbs. cooked minced onions • Sonora Seasoning (see Sonora Spice Blend Recipe). Makes 1 portion. Equals 1 cup cooled starch/grain/beans-legumes.*

Serving amount: 1 cup cooked starch/grain/beans-legumes

Starch/Grains & Beans/Legumes

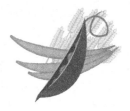

Shrimp & Bean Salad

1. Mix cooked or canned beans, tomato, onion, and cooked cleaned shrimp.
2. Mix vinegar, oil, sweetener (optional), cilantro, basil, and tarragon.
3. Coat beans and shrimp.
4. Cool in refrigerator to season.
5. Serve on salad greens.

- *2 tsp. vinegar • 1 tbs. olive oil*
- *1/8 tsp. dried cilantro • 1/8 tsp. dried basil*
- *1/8 tsp. dried tarragon • 8 ozs. white beans*
- *1/4 cup plum tomato, diced*
- *1/4 cup chopped onion*
- *4 ozs. small shrimp, cooked • 1 cup salad greens. Makes 1 portion. Equals 1 cup cooked starch/ grain/beans-legumes, 4 ozs. protein, 12 ozs or 1 1/2 cups vegetables*

Serving amount: 4 ozs. protein, 1 cup cooked

Split Pea Soup

1. Place all ingredients in a sauce pan and simmer 1 hour.

- *1 cup cooked split peas • 1 tbs. dried celery*
- *1/2 cup chopped carrot • 1 tbs dried celery.*
- *Herbes de Provence spice blend (see Spice Blend Recipe) Makes 1 portion.*

Serving amount: 1 cup cooked starch/grain/ beans-legumes, 1/2 cup starchy vegetable

Vegetable Soup With White Beans

1. Sautee onions and garlic
2. Add other vegetables to pan.
3. Cook until tender. Add water if vegetables get too dry.
4. In a saucepan or microwavable bowl, combine beans and other ingredients. Boil.
5. Add cooked vegetables and simmer.

- *1 cup cooked white or cannellini beans*
- *1 1/2 cup stewed tomatoes • 1/2 cup shredded cabbage • 1/2 cup diced onion • 1/4 cup diced celery • 1/4 cup diced green pepper • 1 cup water*
- *Italian seasoning blend (see Spice Blend Recipes)*
- *Makes 2 portions. Each portion equals 1/2 cup starch/grain/beans-legumes, 1 1/2 cup vegetable.*

Serving amount: 1/2 cup cooked starch/ grain, 12 ozs. or 1 1/2 cups vegetables

Starchy Vegetables

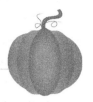

Acorn Squash Puree

1. Put 1/2 cup acorn squash in the blender.
2. Blend until pureed. 3. You can heat up or serve cold. You could also do this with carrots and onions mixed.

• *4ozs. acorn squash • cinnamon • vanilla flavoring • water*

Serving amount: 4 ozs. or 1/2 cup starchy vegetable

Acorn/Winter Squash

1. Cut them in half, remove the seeds, (save to plant).
2. sprinkle cinnamon and sweetener (and extracts if you like per previous recipe) inside the hollowed out space. Then turn upside down and bake them in a 375 oven on a sprayed pan. The skins on. The skins get shinny and pretty. They take a good long while, 45 minutes or more. Should be tender when pierced with toothpick or the like.You can then scrape out the yellow meat, weight and measure and put back into the shell if you like.

• *4 ozs. or 1/2 cup acorn or winter squash*

Serving amount: 4 ozs. or 1/2 cup starchy vegetable

Asparagus Steamed With Cheese

1. Wash fresh asparagus.
2. Cut tips and main part.
3. Discard last 2 inches of stem. Steam in large bowl for 8 minutes in microwave or on stove.
4. Measure 2 ozs. Velveeta cheese or Cheezewiz or other hard cheese.
5. Slice in small chunks to cover steamed asparagus.
6. Cover. Let sit 5 to 10 minutes until cheese is melted.

• *8 to 16 oz. fresh asparagus • 2 oz. homogonize cheese spread without wheat or whey or hard chees*

Serving amount: 8 ozs. or 1 cup vegetable, 2 ozs. cheese or 1 full protein

Starchy Vegetables

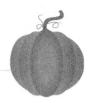

Beets, Cooked

Put them in a small amount of boiling water, cover tightly, and simmer slowly till they are tender to the touch of the finger. Don't pierce them with a fork until they are done. They will take from 30 to 45 minutes. Plunge the cooked beets into cold water. As soon as you can handle them, slip the skins off. Beets may also be baked in the oven at 325 degrees F for an hour. Serving ideas: Serve with roast of pork or grilled pork chops.

• *8 beets* • *1 tsp. lemon juice* • *salt* • *pepper*
• *non-aerosol oil mist*

Serving amount: 4 ozs. or 1/2 cup starchy vegetable

Beets with Spices

Combine ingredients, heat and serve. Heat and serve.

• *1/2 cup canned beets* • *sweetener (optional)* •
allspice • *cloves* • *nutmeg*

Serving amount: 4 ozs. or 1/2 cup starchy vegetable

Butternut Squash I

1. Slice 2 whole washed butternut squashes in half the long way.
2. Place all four halves, sliced-side-down on a cookie sheet.
3. Bake at 400 degrees for 20 minutes, or until the skin is crispy, and the sliced sides are caramelized. May also be microwaved for an easy way to peel after cooking. Microwave 7 minutes at power 7.
4. Slice bulb off of butternut squash end. Slice butternut squash into 1 inch slices. Take vegetable out of skin. Mash butternut squash or cut into small chunks. Measure 1/2 cup for each portion. Makes 4 portions. Each portion equals 1/2 cup starchy vegetable.

• *2 whole butternut squash*

Serving amount: 4 ozs. or 1/2 cup starchy vegetable

Starchy Vegetables

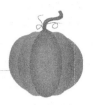

Butternut Squash II - Winter Squash Mashed

1. Seed and quarter squash. Method I: Pressure Cooker–Place the cooking rack in the pressure cooker in order to keep the squash out of the liquid. Add the water. Place the squash on the rack. Close the cover securely. Place the pressure regulator on the vent. Cook at 15 POUNDS for 8 minutes (start timing when the regulator begins to rock). Immerse the pressure cooker in or under running cold water to stop the cooking. Remove the squash. Remove the rack. Discard the remaining water. Cool the squash. Remove and discard the skin. Mash the squash with the sweetener, butter, vinegar and mustard. Season to taste salt and pepper. Return to the pressure cooker. Cook over medium heat until hot. Serve. Method II: Microwave- Place squash onplate and microwave for 2 minutes on high. Remove squash from microwave. Slice off top and bottom and cut into large chunks, removing seeds from bottom portion. Place in a microwave- proof container with about 1/2 inch of water, cover and microwave on high until squash is extremely soft. Peel away the skin (mind your fingers!) and place squash in a large mixing bowl. Mash the squash and beat it together with the sweetener, butter, vinegar and mustard. Season to taste with salt and pepper. Reheat in microwave before serving.

• *1 1/2 cups water ~ 1 tb. vinegar* • *1 2-lb butternut squash seeded and quartered (skin left on)* • *1 tsp Dijon mustard* • *Salt and ground white pepper*

Serving amount: 4 ozs. or 1/2 cup starchy vegetable

Butternut Squash III - Winter Squash Fajita Chips

1. Cut both ends off the squash with a cleaver; then use a small paring knife to remove the skin. Cut off the bottom of the squash and remove seeds. Slice squash into very thin half-circles and spread in a single layer on baking sheets.
2. Sprinkle with seasoning (or salt, pepper, other spices of your choice).
3. Bake at 450 F for about 15 minutes, taking care not to burn squash slices.
4. Measure 1/2 cup portion and serve. This works with other kinds of squash, though not as well, and with rutabagas and turnips. May also be cooked in the oven broiler.

• *2 whole butternut squash*

Serving: 1/2 cup starchy vegetable

Starchy Vegetables

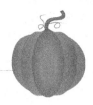

Butternut Squash IV - Winter Squash Roasted or Baked

1. Cut in half lengthwise. Remove seeds. 2. Place on shallow, microwave-safe dish, skin side up.
3. Add small amount of water to bottom of dish.
4. Cover with lid.
5. Microwave for 15-20 minutes, depending on size of squash.
6. Cool for 10 minutes.
7. Scoop out squash. Measure 1/2 cup .
8. Serve hot or chilled. Serving ideas: Serve hot, topped with measured cheese. Serve cold, mixed with yogurt, sweetener, and abstinent flavorings.

• *2 whole butternut squash*

Serving: 1/2 cup starchy vegetable

Butternut Squash V - Winter Squash with Four Chiles

1. Slice in half.
2. Bake the squash for about an hour at 400 F or microwave on Power 7 for 7 minutes until tender.
3. Leave to cool.
4. Soak the chipotle in boiling water for 5 minutes and drain.
6. Pulverize the ancho in a blender or food processor.
7. Stem and seed the habañero.
8. Place all three chiles in a large pot with 1 cup water.
9. Simmer 20 minutes; remove and discard chipotle and habañero.
10. Scrape squash from rind; whirl in blender or food processor and add to pot.
11. Simmer 10 minutes.
12. Meanwhile, use non-calorie cooking spray and sauté the jalapeños and onions oil.
13. When they are finished, add them to the squash and mix thoroughly.

• *2 large butternut squashl* •*3 pound banana or spaghetti squash* • *1 dried chipotle pepper*
• *1 dried ancho chilel* • *1 fresh habañero or other hot pepper* • *1 small red onion finely chopped*
• *2-3 jalapeño peppers roasted and chopped*
• *3 tbs. olive oil*

Serving amount: 4 ozs. or 1/2 cup starchy vegetable

Starchy Vegetables

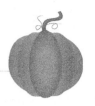

Butternut Squash VI - Winter Squash with Herbs and Spices

1. Peel and cut the squash into pieces.
2. Put in a pan with water, and simmer until just tender. Or microwave on 7 Power for 7 Minutes.
3. Remove squash from pan.
4. Add spices to the liquid, which remains, bring to a boil, return squash to pan, and simmer until squash is very soft.

- *1 medium-sized squash • 1/2 tsp. gound pepper*
- *1/4 tsp. ground cumin • 1/4 tsp. ground ginger*
- *pinch of rosemary • 1 tbs. cider vinegar*

Serving amount: 4 ozs. or 1/2 cup starchy vegetable

Carrot Cinnamon Puree

Measure 1/2 cup cooked carrots. Combine with 1/2 cup soy milk (a 1/4 protein). Mix ingredients in glass blender. Add sufficient boiling water to blend. Blender.

- *3 large raw carrots cut small • 1/2 cup soy milk*
- *salt • ginger • cinnamon • pepper and sweetener*
- *boiling water*

Serving amount: 4 ozs. or 1/2 cup starchy vegetable

Carrot Shredded with Tofu Muffins or Loaf - Dairy-Free - Muffins VI

1. Lightly cook shredded carrot and other vegetables by boiling or in microwave or in small loaf pan by baking a few minutes.
2. Chop tofu fine.
3. Blend tofu, egg whites, shredded carrots and other vegetables together in a blender. You will have a batter
4. Spray muffin tins or loaf pan with non-aerosol oil mist. 5. Pour batter into muffin tins or loaf pan so that they are about 1/2 full.
6. Bake at 325 degrees about 20-30 minutes. Microwave on medium about 8 minutes. Makes 1 portions. Each portion equals 4 ozs. protein, 1/2 cup starchy vegetable, 1 1/2 cups vegetable

- *4 large raw carrots cut small & shredded to make 1/2 cup • 2 ozs. tofu • 2 egg whites*
- *1 1/2 cups zucchini or yellow squash • ginger*
- *cinnamon • Swedish Spice Blend (see Spice Blend Recipes) • sweetener (optional)*
- *boiling water*

Serving amount: 4 ozs. protein, 4 ozs. or 1/2 cup starchy vegetable, 1 1/2 cup cooked vegetable, non-aerosol oil mist

Starchy Vegetables

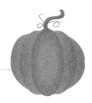

Kabocha Squash Gingered

1. Pour the water into a large, heavy saucepan.
2. Set as many chunks of kabocha, skin side down, as will fit in the water. Sprinkle half the sliced ginger on top. Add the remaining chunks of squash and top with the remaining ginger. Bring the water to a boil. Cover and cook over medium heat until the squash is fork-tender but still firm, 8 to 1 2 minutes. You can remove pieces as they become tender. To prevent scorching, be sure to check every few minutes and replenish water if needed.

- *1 whole kabocha squash. Kabocha looks much like a buttercup squash except for its "navel" (opposite the stem end), which has no bump. The attractive rind, with its dark green and bright orange stripes, need not be peeled-just trim off any unsightly rough spots. You'll need your heaviest chef's knife to hack the kabocha into pieces.*
  - *2 tbs. sliced ginger root*

Serving amount: 4 ozs. or 1/2 cup starchy vegetable

Pumpkin Custard

1. Whisk together first 5 ingredients.
2. Pour into 4 individual oven proof glass bowls.
3. Sprinkle with nutmeg.
4. Put bowls in a cake pan and pour boiling water around the bowls to about 1 inch from top of bowls.
5. Bake at 350 degrees for 45 minuts or until firm. Makes 2 portions. Each portion equals 1 protein, 1 cup dairy, 1/2 cup starchy vegetable.

- *4 eggs beaten* • *2 cups of scalded fat-free milk*
- *1 cup canned 100% pumpkin* • *1 tsp. vanilla flavoring or non-alcohol maple flavoring, nutmeg*
- *sweetener (optional)*

Serving amount: 1 protein, 1 cup dairy, 1/2 cup starchy vegetable

Starchy Vegetables

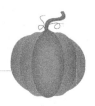

Pumpkin Muffins or Sweet Potato Tofu Muffins or Loaf - Dairy-Free - Muffins VII

1. Mix and stir egg whites, tofu and pumpkin or sweet potato with cinnamon until smooth and well blended.
2. Bake in a loaf pan or muffin tin at 325 degrees for 20 minutes.

• *1/2 cup canned 100% pumpkin* • *2 ozs. tofu* • *2 egg whites* • *1 1/2 cups zucchini or yellow squash* • *ginger* • *cinnamon* • *Swedish Spice Blend (see Spice Blend Recipes) or spices to taste* • *sweetener (optional)* • *boiling water*

Serving amount: 4 ozs. protein, 4 ozs. or 1/2 cup starchy vegetable, 1 1/2 cup cooked vegetable, non-aerosol oil mist

Pumpkin Refritos

1. Place the ancho chile in a small saucepan and cover with water.
2. Bring to a boil.
3. Reduce heat and simmer until chile is soft, about 10 minutes.
4. Remove the chile from the liquid. When it is cool enough to handle, stem the chile, split it open, and scrape out the seeds.
5. Place the pumpkin in a food processor and add the chile, cumin, salt, and cayenne pepper.
6. Process until smooth, stopping to scrape down the sides of the bowl.
7. Transfer to an oven-proof dish and bake at 350° until the top is crusty. Makes manh 1/2 cup starchy vegetable portions.

• *1 dried ancho chile* • *1-2 cans pumpkin* • *1/4 teaspoon ground cumin* • *1 teaspoon salt, plus more to taste* • *scant pinch cayenne pepper*

Serving amount: 4 ozs. or 1/2 cup starchy vegetable

Pumpkin Souffle Pudding

1. Heat 1/2 cup canned pumpkin with spices.
2. Serve as heated side-dish vegetable or as meal pudding.

• *1/2 cup uncooked canned "100% pure pumpkin"* • *1 cup plain yogurt* • *nutmeg and cinnamon to taste*

Serving amount: 4 ozs. or 1/2 cup starchy vegetable

Starchy Vegetables

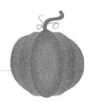

Pumpkin Tart With Soymilk & Oat Crust

1. Set a rack in the middle of the oven and preheat the oven to 375 degrees. Lightly oil a 9-inch tart pan with a removeable bottom or thoroughly grease a 9-inch pie plate. Set aside.

2. To prepare the crust, set the oat bran, oatmeal, cinna¬mon, and salt in the bowl of a food processor. Pulse until the mixture resembles coarse meal, stopping and scraping down the bowl as needed. Transfer to a medium-sized bowl.

3. In a measuring cup, whisk together the oil and water and no alcohol maple flavoring. Pour the liquid into the dry ingredients and blend thoroughly with a fork until the mixture forms a soft dough. Press the mixture into the prepared pan or plate. Crimp the edges if using a pie plate. Bake for 10 minutes. Set on a rack to cool.

4. To prepare the filling, blend the soymilk and arrowroot (an alternative to flour or cornstarch) in the food processor until the arrowroot is completely dissolved and the mixture is smooth, about 15 seconds. Add all of the remaining ingredients. Process until thoroughly blended and smooth, stopping and scraping down the work bowl as needed.

5. Pour the mixture into the crust and smooth the top with a spatula. Bake until the crust is lightly browned and the outside inch of the filling is set, about 35 minutes. Do not be concerned if the center is still soft; it will firm up as the pie cools.

6. Remove from the oven and set on the rack. Cool to room temperature and then refrigerate until completely chilled, about 3 hours. Serve chilled or at room temperature. Leftovers may be refrigerated for up to 3 days. This pumpkin tart has no compromise on flavor and stands up to any traditional. Makes 4 portions. Each portion equals 4 ozs. starchy vegetable, 2 ozs. dairy or protein, 2 tbs. starch & 1.75 ozs. starch/grain = 2 ozs. starch/grain, 1 tbs oil.

• *For the filling: l cup soymilk • 1/4 cup arrowroot • 1 can (16 ounces) solid-pack pumpkin • 2 tbs. no alcohol maple flavoring • 1 tbs. grated fresh ginger • 1 1/2 tsps. ground cinnamon • 1/2 tsp. salt • 1/4 tsp. freshly grated nutmeg • 1/8 tsp. ground cloves.*
• *For the crust: non-aerosol oil mist for preparing tart pan or pie plate • 1/2 cup dry oat bran • 1/4 cup dry rolled oats • 1/2 tsp. ground cinnamon pinch of salt • 1/8 cup oil • 1/8 cup water • 1 tbs. no alcohol maple flavoring*

Serving amount: 4 ozs. or 1/2 cup starchy vegetable, 2 ozs. dairy or protein, 2 tbs. starch & 1.75 ozs. starch/grain = 2 ozs.

Starchy Vegetables

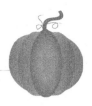

Rutabaga

Peel raw rutabaga with peeler. Carefully poke holes in rutabaga, by stabbing with a fork. Wrap with plastic wrap or moist paper towel. Microwave for 5-7 minutes. Remove from microwave. Let cool for 10 minutes. Leave plastic wrap on to steam while cooling. Remove wrap. Dice rutabaga into small cubes. Measure 1/2 cup and serve.

- *1 fresh rutabaga*

Serving amount: 4 ozs. or 1/2 cup starchy vegetable

Spaghetti Squash I - Winter Squash a la Gorgonzola

1. Split spaghetti squash lengthwise and remove seeds.
2. Place flat side of squash down in amicrowave dish with about ½ inch water andcover.
3. Cook on high for approximately 15-30 minutes. Squash is done when tender but not mushy to the touch. Squash may also be cooked in microwave on Power 7 for 7 minutes.
4. Loosen strands with a fork.
5. Measure out 1/2 cup of the cooked squash.
6. Add remaining ingredients, and microwave until cheese is melted.

7. Save remaining spaghetti squash to make spaghetti squash and cheese dish again soon.

- *1 whole spaghetti squash (winter squash)*
- *1 1/2 ozs. gorgonzola or bleu cheese*
- *1/2 ounce Parmesan or Romano cheese*
- *salt and pepper*

Serving amount: 1 protein, 4 ozs. or 1/2 cup

Spaghetti Squash II - Winter Squash Hawaiian Style

1. Split spaghetti squash lengthwise and remove seeds.
2. Place flat side of squash down in a microwave dish with about ½ inch water andcover.
3. Cook on high for approximately 15-30 minutes. Squash is done when tender butnot mushy to the touch. Squash may also be cooked in microwave on Power 7 for 7minutes.
4. Loosen strands with a fork. 5. Measure out 1/2 cup of the cooked squash.
5. Toss cooked squash with ham and soynuts

- *3 ozs. cooked, diced ham • 1 oz. soy nuts*
- *1/2 cup spaghetti squash (winter squash)*
- *1/2 teaspoon cinnamon*

Serving amount: 4 ozs. protein, 4 ozs. or 1/2 cup starchy vegetable

Starchy Vegetables

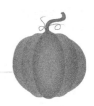

Spaghetti Squash III with Goat Cheese

1. Heat oven to 400 degrees. Prick squash in several places and bake 45 minutes until tender. Squash may also be cooked in microwave - 7 minutes at Power 7.
2. Allow to cool slightly. Cut in half, lengthwise, and scoop out seeds. Pull out squash strands from each side with a fork.
3. Transfer squash without strands to a container for storage.
4. Measure 1/2 cup squash and mix with 2ozs. goat cheese.
5. Reheat spaghetti squash with goat cheese mix in mocrowave or oven.
6. Scoop and serve mix with a scooper or large tablespoon to shape.
7. Serve hot or cold.

- *1 whole spaghetti squash (winter squash)*
- *2 ozs. goat cheese* • *salt and pepper*

Turnip Fries

Heat oven to 425° F. Cut turnips into 2" x 1/2" sticks. Place on a foil-lined pan. Spray with zero-calorie butter spray. Sprinkle with salt and chili powder. Turn with spatula to coat. Spread out in a single layer. Roast fries 30 minutes, turning halfway through cooking time for even browning. Measure 1 cup and serve.

- *4 turnips, trimmed and peeled (about 1 1/4 pounds)* • *non-aerosol oil mist* • *1 teaspoon salt* • *1/2 teaspoon chili powder*

Serving amount: 4 ozs. or 1/2 cup starchy vegetable

Turnip Strips, Roasted

Microwave the turnip for about 10 minutes. Peel and slice the turnip into thin pieces and roast, sprinkling with 1 tsp. olive oil or zero-calorie cooking spray. (1/2 c. if rutebega; 1 c if white turnip)

- *1 cup peeled turnip* • *non-aerosol oil mist*

Serving amount: 4 ozs. or 1/2 cup starchy vegetable

Turnips And Rutabagas, Baked

1. Peel turnips and rutabagas thoroughly andscrub them.
2. Spray with zero calorie butter flavoredcooking spray and poke holes in vegetablesto permit cooking.
3. Wrap in foil but leave an opening on top.
4. Bake at 275 degrees for about 1.5-2.0 hours until browned and soft.
5. Or microwave on 8 power for 8-9minutes. Makes 1 portion of 1/2 cup starchyvegetable.

- *1/4 cup turnips* • *1/4 cup rutabagas*

Serving amount: 4 ozs. or 1/2 cup starchy

Cooked Vegetables

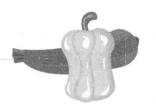

Artichokes, Steamed With Curry Dipping Sauce

1. Cut the tops and stem end off the artichoke.
2. Steam artichoke for 45 minutes.
3. Measure 1 cup.
4. Mix curry powder into allowable portion of mayonnaise until it reaches the level of spiciness that suits you.

- *1 artichoke* • *1 tsp. mayonnaise*
- *1/2 tsp. curry powder*

Serving amount: 4 ozs. starchy vegetable or 1/2 cup starchy vegetable, 1 tsp. oil

Asparagus, Broiled, Roasted o Steamed

1. Wash asparagus. Trim if necessary. Peel with a peeler so long strings are removed.
2. If Broiling, place in casserole dish. Spray with zero-calorie butter spray.
3. Place garlic slices randomly between asparagus pieces (the more garlic, the better - minced garlic works fine also). Sprinkle lightly with salt.
4. Broil in oven for 10-15 minutes, or until slightly browned and crispy.
5. If roasting, place in a roaster oven in a glass plate. Cook for 15 minutes at 325 degrees.
6. Shake pan once or twice during baking time. Roasting brings out the natural sweetness in most vegetables, and intensifies their flavor.If steaming or boiling, use steamer and steam for 10 minutes. Measure 1 cup and serve.

- *1cup asparagus* • *non-aerosol oil mist*
- *2 -3 garlic cloves thinly sliced*
- *1/4 tsp. salt*

Serving amount: 8 ozs. or 1 cup vegetable

Cooked Vegetables

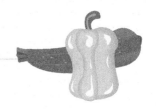

Babaganoush Eggplant Dip for Raws

1. Cut up ripe Japanese eggplants, about 4-5 (it is sweeter than regular).
2. Put into clear plastic produce bag and poke a hole in it and nuke for about 8 minutes until mushy.
3. Put into the food processor with garlic powder, onion powder, salt and pepper to taste, lemon juice.
4. Clean 1 head cauliflower.
5. Cook cauliflower the same way in the bag and nuke until mushy.
6. Put all veggies into the food processor and make babaganoush mush. Weigh out 8 oz and use for a dip.

- *4-5 Japanese eggplants • 1 head cauliflower*
- *2 tsp. garlic powder • 1 tsp. onion powder*
- *1 tbs. lemon juice.*

Serving amount: 8 ozs. or 1 cup vegetable

Beef Vegetable Soup or Stew

1. Place 5 cups water in a large pot of 3 qt. saucepan or slow cooker.
2. Boil the beef piece slowly in the water for 15 to 20 minutes.
3. When beef is almost cooked, add 1/4 cup quality tomato sauce to the beef broth cooking.
4. Continue to simmer. Meanwhile, wash, clean, pare, cut and weigh vegetables to equal 12 ozs. (1 1/2 cups vegetable.).
5. Remove beef from beef-tomato stock.
6. Set aside to cool a bit.
7. Place prepared vegetables in beef-tomato stock to cook for 15 to 20 minutes.
8. Meanwhile, cut beef into small pieces.
9. Weigh beef to measure 4 ozs.
10. Put beef pieces back in with the vegetable-tomato-beef stock.
11. Add 1 cup extra water if stock has boiled down. 12. Cook an additional 5 minutes.

- *4 oz. beef (no bone) • 5 cups water*
- *1/4 cup quality tomato sauce • 8 ozs. fresh green beans • 6 ozs. fresh green pepper • 2 ozs. red spanish onion .*

Serving amount: 12 ozs. or 1 1/2 cup vegetable, 4 ozs. Protein

Cooked Vegetables

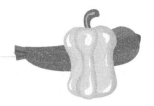

Beet Greens, Collard Greens, Kale, Swiss Chard, or Spinach, Braised, Steamed or Baked

1. Wash the greens well several times.
2. Place in a heavy kettle. Cover tightly.
3. Let them wilt over medium heat.
4. Toss with a fork several times to mix the top greens with the bottom greens.
5. When they are just wilted and tender, remove them and drain thoroughly, then chop and drain some more.
6. Measure 12 ozs or 1 1/2 cup.
7. Top with lemon juice, salt, pepper, and dash of nutmeg. These are pungent and pleasing to the palate.

- *1 - 2 pounds beet greens or other greens*
- *non-aerosol oil mist • 1 tsp. lemon juice*
- *salt*
- *pepper • dash of nutmeg*

Serving amount: 12 ozs. or 1 1/2 cup vegetable

Beet Greens - With Lemon & Nutmeg

1. Wash the greens well several times.
2. Place in a heavy kettle. Cover tightly.
3. Let them wilt over medium heat.
4. Toss with a fork several times to mix thetop greens with the bottom greens.
5. When they are just wilted and tender,remove them and drain thoroughly, thenchop and drain some more.
6.Measure 1 cup.
7. Top with lemon juice, salt, pepper, anddash of nutmeg. These are pungent andpleasing to the palate.

- *1 - 2 pounds beet greens • 1 tsp. lemon juice*
- *salt • pepper • dash of nutmeg*

Cooked Vegetables

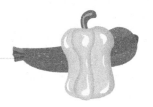

Beets With Spices, Baked or Boiled

1. Put beets (canned or fresh) in a small amount of boiling water, cover tightly, and simmer slowly till they are tender to the touch of the finger. Don't pierce them with a fork until they are done.
2. Fresh beets will take from 30 to 45 minutes to cook. Plunge the cooked beets into cold water.
3. As soon as you can handle them, slip the skins off.
4. Beets may also be baked in the oven at 325 degrees F for an hour.
5. Beets can also be microwaved to remove skins. Microwave 8 power for 8 minutes. Makes 2 portions. Each portion equals 4 ozs. or 1/2 cup. Top with spices and allowable portion of fat and toss. Serving ideas: Serve with roast of pork or grilled pork chops.

- *8 fresh beets or 1 cup canned beets* • *1 tbs lemon juice* • *sweetener (optional)* • *allspice* • *cloves* • *nutmeg*

Serving amount: 4 ozs. or 1/2 cup starchy vegetable

Bell Peppers, Roasted Over Open Flame

1. Over an open flame on the stove, or under a broiler, roast peppers until skins are charred on all sides.
2. Place in a paper or plastic bag and seal bag. Let peppers steam 10 minutes.

3. When peppers are cool enough to handle, peel, seed and cut into 1/3- inch-wide strips.
4. Transfer to a glass dish. Measure 1 cup and serve.

- *4 bell peppers whole* • *any color*
- *non-aerosol oil mist*

Serving amount: 8 ozs. or 1 cup vegetable

Bell Peppers, Roasted or Baked

1. Over an open flame on the stove, or under a broiler, roast peppers until skins are charred on all sides.
2. Place in a paper or plastic bag and seal bag.
3. Let peppers steam 10 minutes.
4. When peppers are cool enough to handle, peel, seed and cut into 1/3- inch-wide strips.
5. Transfer to a glass dish.
6. For Roasted Peppers, spray glass dish with zero-calorie butter spray or no spray needed.
7. Place peppers (any color) in glass dish.
8. Roast in oven or roaster oven at 325 degrees for 40 minutes. Measure 1 1/2 cup and serve.

- *4 bell peppers whole* • *any color, zero-calorie butter spray (olive oil flavored)*

Serving amount: 12 ozs. or 1 1/2 cup vegetable

Cooked Vegetables

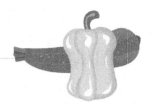

Broccoli, Boiled, Steamed, Tangy or with Lemon Sauce

1. Since broccoli florets cook more quickly than stems, peel the stalks down to the white flesh and cut into short lengths. Cut off hard ends and remove outer leaves.
2. Soak for 30 minutes in salted water (optional).
3. In boiling, cook stalks in boiling, salted water for about 5 minutes.
4. Then, add the florets and cook another 5 minutes. If steaming, steam for 12-14 minutes, or until just tender, being careful not to overcook.
5. Drain well.
6. Measure out 1 cup.
7. If Tangy style, add 2 tablespoons mustard (preferably English mustard) • 2 teaspoons soy sauce • 1 teaspoon non-aerosol oil mist. If with lemon juice, add 2 tbs lemon juice.

• *8 ozs. or 1 cup vegetable, 4 tbs. no sugar condiment (mustard, optional), 1 tbs. lemon juice*

Serving amount: 8 ozs. or 1 cup vegetable

Broccoli Souffle or Crustless Quiche

1. Puree, or finely chop, cooked broccoli.
2. Beat eggs in a bowl until thoroughly mixed.
3. Spray shallow glass or foil casserole dish with zero-calorie butter spray
4. Pour beaten eggs into baking dish.
5. Fold in broccoli until mixed with eggs.
6. Season with nutmeg and black pepper.
7. Bake for 15 minutes at 325 degrees until eggs are set or microwave on high for 2-3 minutes until eggs are set.

• *2 eggs • 1 cup broccoli • non-aerosol oil mist* • *salt, pepper*

Serving amount: 12 ozs. or 1 1/2 cup vegetab,e 2 eggs or 1 full protein

Broccoli With Lemon

1. Cut off hard ends and remove outer leaves.
2. Soak for 30 minutes in salted water.
3. Place in pot of 1 pint boiling water (salted).
4. Stalks down.
5. Remove and drain.
6. Chop garlic very fine and mix thru.
7. Measure out 1 cup and add lemon and margarine.

• *1 1/2 cups or 12 ounces broccoli • garlic* • *1 tbs. lemon juice*

Serving amount: 12 ozs. or 1 1/2 cup vegetable

Cooked Vegetables

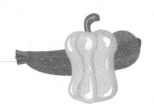

Brocolette or Broccoli Rabe With Garlic & Tofu

1. Brocolette is a cross between broccoli and kale. It has small long stalks and leggy florets. All of it may be eaten. It is tender when cooked. It has the taste of broccoli.
2. Cut a bunch of brocolette and place in a microwavable bowl or a steamer. 3. Cut the tofu into chunks and toss in. 4. Cook the brocolette with a lid on top for about 8 minutes on power 8 in the microwave, or about 15 minutes in a steamer. Brocollette is easy to prepare with a protein or with a seasoning blend.

- *1 1/2 cups or 12 ozs. broccolette* • *4 ozs. tofu*
- *1 tb.lemon juice* • *garlic powder or 1 clove garlic minced*

Serving amount: 12 ozs. or 1 1/2 cup vegetable

Cabbage and Green Peppers

1. In a microwave-safe, covered dish, microwave the ground round, oregano, garlic, parsley, ginger, mustard, celery, onion, and green pepper for 2 minutes.
2. Stir the mixture, being careful not to burn yourself on the steam. Microwave on high for another 2 to 3 minutes, or until the meat is no longer pink.
3. Drain any fat residue or dab the beef mixture with a paper towel.
4. Heat the steamed cabbage in the microwave on high for 30 seconds to 1 minute to warm it to serving temperature.
5. Toss the chopped, raw tomato with the ground round mixture and spoon it over the warmed cabbage. Sprinkle the dried basil over the top of the dish and serve.

- *4.5 ozs. uncooked beef ground round*
- *1/8 tsp. dried oregano* • *1/4 tsp. minced, dried garlic (or 1/2 clove minced fresh garlic)*
- *1/4 tsp. dried parsley* • *Dash of dried ginger*
- *Dash of dried mustard* • *2 tbs. chopped celery*
- *2 tbs. chopped onion*
- *1/2 cup chopped green pepper*
- *1/2 cup steamed cabbage,shredded or rough chopped*
- *1/2 cup medium peeled, chopped tomato*
- *1/4 tsp. dried basil*

Serving amount: 1 protein, 12 ozs. or 1 1/2 cup vegetable

Cooked Vegetables

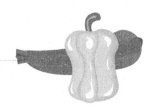

Cabbage Fried - Pennsylvania Dutch Style

1. Add cabbage to non-aerosol oil mist in frying pan.
2. Cook on high for 5 minutes to lightly browned.
3. Turn heat down.
4. Cover cabbage and cook, tossing lightly occasionally, for about 20 minutes.

• *2-3 cups green cabbage*

Serving amount: 12 ozs. or 1 1/2 cup vegetable, non-aerosol oil mist

Cabbage Kimchee - Thai Cabbage

1. Salt the cabbage and toss. 2. Place in colander. 3. Place weights on top. I do this in the morning and then later in the afternoon I do the rest. 4. Take the cabbage add red pepper flakes, finely chopped fresh ginger, sweetener and rice vinegar. Depending on how hot and spicy you like your food that is how much of the red pepper flakes and ginger you should add.

• *cabbage* • *red pepper flakes*
• *ginger-fresh & chopped* • *sweetener (optional)*
• *1/4-1/2 cup vinegar*

Serving amount: 12 ozs. or 1 1/2 cup vegetable

Collard Greens - Braised

1. Spray skillet with non-aerosol oil mist.
2. Sauté garlic over med-hi heat. When tender, add greens.
3. Stir for 2-3 minutes, then add enough water to almost cover the greens.
4. Stir occasionally. When greens are tender and bright green, and some of the water has boiled off, add a splash of vinegar and pepper.
5. Measure 1 1/2 cup and serve. Variation: Also sauté with 1 medium yellow onion or cut portion in half.

---

1 lb. collard greens, washed, torn, and with stems removed • *2 large cloves garlic, minced* • *non-aerosol oil mist* • *vinegar* • *pepper*

Serving amount: 12 ozs. or 1 1/2 cup vegetable, non-aerosol oil mist

Cooked Vegetables

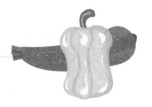

Eggplant - Basic Grilled or Roasted

1. Heat oven to 425° F.
2. Cut the eggplant on all sides with deep slashes and place in a baking pan.
3. Roast until soft, 30 to 40 minutes.
4. Set aside until cool enough to handle, about 15 minutes
5. Peel eggplant and coarsely chop.
6. Place in a medium bowl.
7. Spray with non-aerosol oil mist.
8. Add garlic, salt, pepper and parsley.
9. Measure 1 1/2 cup and serve.

• *1 eggplant or 2 italian eggplants* • *non-aerosol oil mist* • *2 garlic cloves, pushed through a press* • *1/2 tsp. salt , freshly ground black pepper to taste* • *chopped fresh parsley to taste*

Serving amount: 12 ozs. or 1 1/2 cup vegetable, non-aerosol oil mist

Eggplant Dip for Raws - Babaganoush

1. Cut up ripe Japanese eggplants, about 4-5 (it is sweeter than regular).
2. Put into clear plastic produce bag and poke a hole in it and nuke for about 8 minutes until mushy.
3. Put into the food processor with garlic powder, onion powder, salt and pepper to taste, lemon juice.
4. Clean 1 head cauliflower.
5. Cook cauliflower the same way in the bag and nuke until mushy.
6. Put all veggies into the food processor and make babaganoush mush. Weigh out 8 oz and use for a dip.

• *4-5 Japanese eggplants* • *1 head cauliflower*
• *2 tsp. garlic powder* • *1 tsp. onion powder*
• *1 tbs. lemon juice.*

Serving amount: 8 ozs. or 1 cup vegetable

Cooked Vegetables

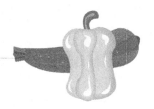

Eggplant Ratatouille I

1. Coat skillet with non-aerosol oil mist.
2. Cook onions & garlic in the vinegar and water, then add green peppers, cook a bit, add zucchini, cook a bit more, then add rest of ingredients.
3. Add water and/or vinegar as necessary to keep it from burning.

• *1 large eggplant* • *peeled and cubed* • *1 large zucchini sliced and peeled* • *tomato paste to taste* • *green peppers, cored and de-seeded* • *onions, peeled and sliced into rounds then into quarters or use onion seasoning* • *fresh garlic, chopped or just peeled* • *vinegar* • *water as needed to keep mixture from burning* • *salt & pepper to taste* • *oregano* • *basil* • *bay leaf*

Serving amount: 12 ozs. or 1 1/2 cup vegetable, non-aerosol oil mist

Eggplant Rattouille II

1. Season all of the veggies with oregano or any Italian seasoning, salt and pepper I take the eggplant slice it into quarters, spray a cookie sheet with non-aerosol oil mist.
2. Bake in oven until it begins to get tender. In the meantime cut up remaining vegetables and sauté them in a large pot sprayed with non-aerosol oil mist. Once they are tender mix them with the eggplant and can of crusted tomatoes.
3. Put the mixture into a casserole dish and bake until the tomatoes began to bubble and all of the veggies are tender.
4. You can measure out 12 ozs. of veggies for lunch or your required amount for dinner.

• *2 eggplants* • *2 yellow squash* • *2 zucchini*
• *1 green pepper* • *1 red pepper* • *1 onion*
• *2 cloves garlic* • *1 can of crushed tomatoes*
• *oregano* • *salt* • *ground pepper*

Serving amount: 12 ozs. or 1 1/2 cup vegetable, non-aerosol oil mist

Cooked Vegetables

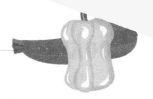

Eggplant Salad, Cold Mediterranean Roasted Eggplant

1. Roast eggplants in the broiler or on grill.
2. Cut into cubes.
3. Add remaining ingredients.

• *Eggplant* • *1 small clove garlic* • *salt to taste*
• *non=aerosol oil mist* • *1 tsp.lemon juice*

Serving amount: 8 ozs. or 1 cup vegetables

Eggplant-Spinach Curry

1. Heat non-aerosol oil mist with half of the mustard seeds in a large saucepan.
2. Add remaining mustard seeds when the cooked seeds begin to pop.
3. Add the garlic and sauté over fairly low heat until it begins to turn golden.
4. Add the spinach, a small amount at a time, stirring occasionally to keep it from scorching. There is less danger of this with frozen spinach, which tends to have quite a bit of water in it. When the spinach wilts, add the eggplant, ginger, jalapeno pepper, turmeric, paprika, coriander, and cumin.
5. Sauté to blend the flavors.
6. Cover and cook over medium-low heat for 15 minutes.
7. Add the tomatoes and season to taste with salt.
8. Cook, uncovered, 5 minutes longer.
9. Garnish with cilantro.

• *non-aerosol oil mist* • *1 tsp. black mustard seeds*
• *12 cloves garlic peeled and coarsely chopped*
• *2 lbs. fresh spinach rinsed dried and finely chopped, (or 1 good-sized package frozen chopped spinach)* • *1 medium eggplant cut into 1/2-inch cubes* • *1-inch piece fresh ginger peeled and grated*
• *1 jalapeno pepper minced* • *1/4 tsp. turmeric*
• *1/4 tsp. paprika* • *1/2 tsp. ground coriander*
• *1/2 tsp. ground cumin* • *1 can chopped tomatoes* • *salt* • *cilantro sprigs for garnish*

Serving amount: 12 ozs. or 1 1/2 cup vegetable, non-aerosol oil mist

French Onions

1. Heat a large casserole or heavy pot and coat with non-aerosol oil mist.
2. Add onions, cover, and simmer over low heat for 2 to 3 hours, stirring thoroughly once every 10 minutes.
3. When onions are a rich brown and very soft, mix in the soy sauce and simmer 10 to 15 minutes more. For best flavor, allow to cool overnight and reheat.

• *non-aerosol oil mist* • *6 medium onions sliced very thin* • *2 tbs. soy sauce*

Serving amount: 12 ozs. or 1 1/2 cup vegetable, non-aerosol oil mist

Vegetables

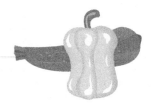

Green Peppers & Onions, Italian Style

1. Put peppers and onions in a deep frying pan with non-aerosol oil mist.
2. Cook on high for 5 minutes to brown lightly.
3. Turn heat down.
4. Cover and cook 20 minutes, tossing lightly.

- *2 to 3 cups cut up green peppers and onions*
- *non-aerosol oil mist*

Serving amount: 12 ozs. or 1 1/2 cup vegetable, non-aerosol oil mist

Greens, Cooked

1. Spray skillet with non-aerosol oil mist.
2. Sauté garlic over med-hi heat. When tender, add greens.
3. Stir for 2-3 minutes, then add enough water to almost cover the greens.
4. Greens may also be boiled or steamed in a small amount of water.
5. Stir occasionally. When greens are tender and bright green, and some of the water has boiled off, add a splash of vinegar and pepper.
6. Measure 1 1/2 cup and serve. Variation: Also sauté with 1 medium yellow onion or cut portion in half.

---

1 lb. greens, washed, torn, and w/ stems removed
- *2 large cloves garlic, minced* • *non-aerosol oil mist* • *vinegar* • *pepper*

Serving amount: 12 ozs. or 1 1/2 cup vegetable, non-aerosol oil mist

Mushrooms, Grilled Portabello 1

1. Remove stems of mushrooms, and wipe them with a damp cloth.
2. Preheat the broiler or grill. Mix vinegar, herbs, and garlic in a bowl.
3. Spray mushrooms with non-aerosol oil mist.
4. Brush mushrooms with the vinegar mixture.
5. Grill or broil the mushrooms 3-5 minutes per side, or until soft and brown.
6. Measure 1 cup and serve.

- *6 medium portabello mushrooms*
- *1 tsp. fresh rosemary or 1/2 tsp. dried rosemary*
- *3 tbs. balsamic vinegar* • *1 tsp. fresh thyme or 1/2 tsp. dried thyme* • *2 cloves garlic thinly sliced*
- *salt and pepper*

Serving amount: 12 ozs. or 1 1/2 cup vegetable, non-aerosol oil mist

Cooked Vegetables

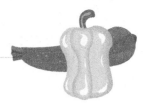

Mushrooms, Grilled Portobello II - Broiled, Sauteed or Steamed

1. Use large caps for broiling. 2. Spray with non-aerosol oil mist. 3. Place on broiler rack, cap side up, about 4 inches from the broiling unit. Broil 2 to 2 1/2 minutes, then turn them over. 4. Add a dash of salt, pepper, and/or Tabasco sauce into each cap. 5. Cook another 2 1/2 minutes. Serving ideas: Top with allowable portion of parsley or dill.

• *1 pound mushrooms • non-aerosol oil mist • salt*
• *pepper • tabasco sauce*

Serving amount: 12 ozs. or 1 1/2 cup vegetable, non-aerosol oil mist

Mushrooms Portobello III With Parmesan Cheese Topping

1. Measure mushrooms.
2. Cook 1 1/2 cups of the big mushroom caps in the non-aerosol oil mist, letting them simmer so they get soft.
3. Measure 1 cup mushrooms.
4. Top with 1 ounce of grated cheese.

• *1 cup portabella mushroom caps*
• *non-aerosol oil mist • 1 oz. grated cheese*

Serving amount: 12 ozs. or 1 1/2 cup vegetable, non-aerosol oil mist, 1/2 protein

Onions I, Cipolline Onions Grilled, Broiled

1. Preheat broiler or grill. If you are using wooden skewers, soak them in water.
2. Measure the oil into a small bowl.
3. Peel onions and cut off both ends. If the onions are more than 1-inch thick, slice them in half.
4. Thread onto skewers.
5. Brush with the oil until thoroughly covered, then sprinkle with salt and pepper.
6. Broil or grill.

• *1-2 lbs cipolline onions • non-aerosol oil mist •*
salt and pepper • skewers

Serving amount: 8 ozs. or 1 cup vegetables

Cooked Vegetables

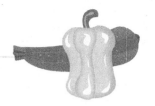

Onions II
Roasted Vidalia

1. Peel the onions and core with a knife or apple corer. Try not to go all the way through, so that you've made sort of a well. (You may need to use a grapefruit spoon to achieve this.)
2. Spray the inside with non-aerosol oil mist. Lightly salt & pepper each onion and wrap in aluminum foil.
3. Place on a moderately hot spot of a grill for 45 minutes to an hour. A knife should go through it like butter. Whatever you do, it'll be good, but perfection is almost black on the bottom where the onion sugars have almost burned & very tender on the inside. This is intended to make 1 8-oz serving.

- *2 medium vidalia onions* • *non-aerosol oil mist*
- *salt and pepper*

Serving amount: 8 ozs or 1 cup vegetable,

Rajas Con Jitomate - Poblanos Chiles

1. Remove the seeds and veins from the chiles and cut them into strips about 1 1/2 inches long and 1/2 inch wide. You may want to substitute anaheim chiles for poblanos–they are milder.
2. Heat non-aerosol oil mist and fry the onions gently, without browning them, until they are soft.
3. Add the chile strips, tomatoes and salt to the onions in the pan.
4. Cook uncovered over a fairly high flame until the vegetables are well seasoned and the liquid has evaporated.

- *8 chiles poblano chiles roasted and peeled*
- *non-aerosol oil mist* • *1 1/2 medium onions thinly sliced* • *1 tsp. salt*
- *2 cans chopped tomatoes drained*

Serving amount: 12 ozs. or 1 1/2 cup vegetable, non-aerosol oil mist

Cooked Vegetables

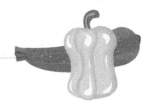

Roasted Vegetables

1. Slice any vegetables thin and lay them out on aluminum foil on a pan. Spray vegetables with non-aerosol oil mist, then lay the slices, cover them with salt, pepper, dill, or any other seasoning that appeals (cinnamon isn't bad – along with some Indian spices), try oregano and thyme, then spray again!!!
2. Roast in oven for 20 minutes or thereabouts – you can tell they are done if the edges start to look burnt!

• *1 1/2 cups vegetables of your choice - zucchini, eggplant, red green or orange peppers, or starchy vegetables like rutabaga* • *non-aerosol oil mist*
• *seasonings*

Serving amount: 12 ozs. or 1 1/2 cup vegetable, non-aerosol oil mist

Spicy Green Peppers

1. Remove stem and seeds from green peppers.
2. Cut into long slices.
3. Heat non-aerosol oil mist in a pan and fry pepper slices until light brown.
4. Remove from pan and add mustard seeds.
5. When mustard seeds begin to pop, add onions; cook 4-5 minutes over medium heat.
6. Add cumin, salt, and cayenne; stir and cook for a few minutes.
7. Return peppers to pot, and 1/2 cup water, and bring to a boil.
8. Simmer 3-4 minutes and serve hot.

• *6 medium sized green peppers* • *2 medium onions* • *finely chopped* • *1 tsp. mustard seeds*
• *1 tb. ground cumin* • *1/2 tsp. cayenne*
• *3 tbs. lemon juice* • *salt to taste*
• *non-aerosol oil mist*

Serving amount: 12 ozs. or 1 1/2 cup vegetable, non-aerosol oil mist

Cooked Vegetables

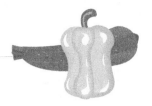

Spinach And Portabello Mushrooms, Sauteed

1. Spray skillet or sauté pan with non-aerosol oil mist.
2. Over medium heat, sauté vegetables and spices until mushrooms are tender, and spinach is heated through.
3. Measure 1 1/2 cup and serve. Variation: Top with grated parmesan cheese as measured portion of protein.

- *2 large portabello mushrooms sliced*
- *1 10-ozs. package frozen chopped spinach, thawed and drained or fresh spinach or kale or greens* • *1/4 tsp. dried basil* • *1/4 tsp. salt*
- *1/4 tsp. black pepper* • *1 clove garlic chopped*
- *non-aerosol oil mist*

Serving amount: 12 ozs. or 1 1/2 cup vegetable, non-aerosol oil mist

String Beans in Garlic Sauce

1. Trim ends off beans and cut in half. In one bowl, combine garlic and chili paste.
2. In another bowl, mix soy sauce, vinegar, and sweetener (optional).
3. Heat wok sprayed with non-aerosol oil mist over medium heat.
4. Add the green beans and stir-fry until they begin to brown. Remove to a bowl.
5. Add scallions to wok, stir-fry quickly, and remove to same bowl.
6. Heat wok sprayed with non-aerosol oil mist again. When it is hot, add garlic/chili paste mixture.
7. Stir for about 12 seconds, then add beans and stir to mix well. 3. Add soy sauce mixture, and stir for a minute. May be prepared ahead and served cold.
8. Quite hot; cut down on the chili paste if you have a low spice tolerance.

- *1 1/2 pounds fresh string beans* • *6 cloves garlic, pressed* • *2 tsp. chili paste w/garlic or 3 tbs. sugar-free ketchup with chili pepper and garlic powder added* • *1 tb. soy sauce* • *1 tb. vinegar*
- *2 tsp. liquid sweetener* • *1 1/2 cups diced scallions* • *non-aerosol oil mist*

Serving amount: 12 ozs. or 1 1/2 cup vegetable, non-aerosol oil mist

Cooked Vegetables

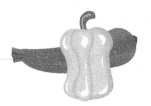

Sun-Dried Tomatoes, Homemade Baked

1. Slice the tomatoes in half vertically, remove seeds, and place face-up on baking sheets.
2. Sprinkle with salt and bake at 400 degrees for 15 minutes.
3. Lower heat to 225 degrees and bake for another 2 1/2 hours; check them after about 2 hours to make sure the bottoms have not burned.
4. When tomatoes are small, shriveled things, put them in plastic containers and add garlic and basil.
5. Cover the sun-dried tomatoes with olive oil, if desired though not necessary.
6. Seal the containers and freeze until ready to use.

• *buckets of fresh flavorful roma tomatoes* • *salt*
• *fresh basil* • *fresh garlic*

Serving amount: 4 ozs. or 1/2 cup vegetable, non-aerosol oil mist

Zucchini Ratatouille III

1. Cover and cook for about 1 hour on very low flame.

• *3 or 4 zucchini in 1 inch chunks*
• *1 large purple onion (purple only for vitamins, any color is ok)*
• *2 very large tomatoes or about 4 plum tomatoes*
• *1 whole box, or about 10 mushrooms*
• *1 green pepper*

Serving amount: 12 ozs. or 1 1/2 cup

Cooked Vegetables with Protein

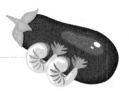

Eggplant Parmesan I

1. Slice eggplant as thin as you can.
2. Lay slices on baking sheets (1 layer only) and sprinkle with ample amounts of paprika, curry, and salt.
3. Spray with non-aerosol oil mist.
4. Dust layers with 1 ozs. Grated pramesan cheese.
5. Bake at 325 degrees for 20 minutes.

• *1 eggplant • paprika • non-aerosol oil mist • 1 oz. grated parmesan cheese • 1 cup crushed tomatoes • 1 tsp. basil • Italian Seasoning Spice Blend (See Spice Blend Recipes)*

Serving amount: 12 ozs. or 1 1/2 cup vegetable, 1 ozs. Cheese or 1/2 protein, non-aerosol oil mist

Eggplant Parmesan II

1. Cut an eggplant up either in rounds or lengthwise. Place in a glass baking dish.
2. Spray with non-aerosol oil mist. 3. Soak the eggplant slices in water for 30-40 minutes.
3. Squeeze the eggplant slices dry of water with paper towels.
4. Layer the eggplant slices with the mozarella cheese and the tomato sauce. Save a few slices of the mozarella to place on top of the baking dish for last few minutes of cooking.
5. Put the baking dish in a 350 oven for 30 minutes.
6. Place the saved mozarella pieces on the eggplant and let cook another 30 minutes.

• *1 eggplant • non-aerosol oil mist • 1/2 tsp. salt • 1/2 jar no sugar tomato sauce • 1 oz. grated parmesan cheese • 1 oz. mozarella cheese*

Serving amount: 12 ozs. or 1 1/2 cup vegetable, 1 protein, non-aerosol oil mist

Cooked Vegetables with Protein

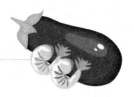

Eggplant with Ricotta and Tomato Sauce

1. Slice eggplant thinly. Measure 8 ozs. or 1 cup eggplant slices.
2. Spray with non-aerosol oil mist, sprinkle with garlic powder, oregano, basil the works.
3. Lay on a cookie sheet or foil.
4. Layer the eggplant slices with 1/2 cup tomato scuce and 2 ozs. ricotta cheese.
5. Turn on the broiler of your oven 6. Broil the eggplant caprese layers for 3-5 minutes.

• *1 eggplant* • *non-aerosol oil mist* • *garlic powder*
• *oregano* • *basil* • *1/2 cup tomato sauce*
• *2 ozs. ricotta cheese*

Serving amount: 12 ozs. or 1 1/2 cup vegetable, 1 protein, non-aerosol oil mist

Lobster and Cauliflower Salad

1. Chop the raw cauliflower into small pieces.
2. Marinate the cauliflower in 1 tbs lemon for 2 hours.
3. Drain.
4. Combine the cauliflower with the cooked and chilled lobster pieces.
5. Add 1 tbs. mustard. Variations: 4 oz. shrimp, or 2 oz. lobster and 1 hard boiled egg, sliced.

• *4 ozs. cooked lobster chunks* • *1 1/2 cups cauliflower, washed and cut into paper-thin slices*
• *1 tbs. mustard*

Serving amount: 12 ozs. or 1 1/2 cup vegetable, 1 protein

Manhattan Clam Chowder - Slow Cooker or Stove Method

1. Open 1 large can of crushed or stewed tomatoes.
2. Open frozen green beans and measure 1cup.
3. Chop 1 cup carrots into small pieces.
4. Open small can of chopped clams. Measure 4 ozs. Add chopped clams forManhattan Clam Chowder.
5. Place crushed tomatoes, green beans,carrots, and clams in a slow cooker or largesaucepan.
6. Cook soup-stew-chowder on slow simmerfor 2 hours.

• *2 cups crushed or stewed tomatoes (1 large can)* • *1 cup water* • *1 cup cooked or uncooked chopped green beans* • *1 cup carrots cut into small pieces* • *4 ozs. chopped clams* • *Herbes de provence (see Spice Blend Recipes). Makes 2 portions. Each portion equals: 2 ozs. protein, 1/2 cup starchy vegetable, 12 ozs or 1 1/2 cup vegetable*

Serving amount: 2 ozs. protein, 1/2 cup starchy vegetable, 12 ozs or 1 1/2 cups vegetables

Cooked Vegetables with Protein

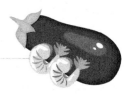

Mixed Grille with Vegetables & Protein

1. Weigh and measure about 16 ozs. vegetables. This will allow for about 4 ozs. water shrinkage in grilling and you can weigh and measure 16 oz (2 c) vegetables after cooking.
2. Weigh & measure about 5-6 oz protein: chicken, salmon, shrimp, catfish, tilapia, Chilean sea bass, London broil, lamb, steak, chicken livers, chops, hamburger, turkey burger, salmon burger, hard tofu.
3. Slice zucchini lengthwise. Slice green, red and yellow peppers into strips. Slice onions into quarters Slice tomatoes into 6ths.
4. Start cooking zucchini and green peppers first, as they take the longest to cook. Remove from grill. Then cook tomatoes and onions. Remove from grill. Then cook protein. 5. Weigh and measure for 12 ozs or 1 1/2 cups vegetables and 4 ozs. protein..

• *5-6 ozs. protein:* • *chicken* • *salmon* • *shrimp* • *catfish* • *tilapia* • *chilean sea bass* • *london broil* • *lamb* • *steak* • *chicken livers* • *chops* • *hamburger* • *turkey burger* • *salmon burger* • *hard tofu.* • *16 ozs. vegetables:* • *zucchini* • *green peppers* • *red peppers* • *yellow peppers* • *onions* • *tomatoes*

Serving amount: 12 ozs. or 1 1/2 cup vegetable, 1 protein

Pork Chop With Sauerkraut

1. Pan fry or broil 4 oz. pork chop. 2. Heat or serve with 1 cup canned sauerkraut. Frying pan or broiler.

• *4 oz. pork chop* • *1 cup sauerkraut*

Serving amount: 8 ozs. or 1 cup vegetable, 4 ozs. protein

Sauerkraut with Frankfurters

1. Buy sauerkraut in the deli cold section or canned sauerkraut or fresh sauerkraut, making sure that there is no sugar listed in the ingredients.
2. Chop 2 beef frankfurters and place in 1 cups sauerkraut.
3. Heat through. Makes 1 protion. Portion equals 4 ozs protein, 1 cup cooked vegetable.

• *8 ozs. no-sugar sauerkraut*
• *2 beef frankfurters*

Serving amount: 4 ozs.protein, 8 ozs. or 1 cup vegetable

Cooked Vegetables with Protein

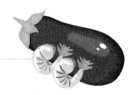

Salmon Stir Fry

1. Open large can of canned salmon, 15 ozs. 2. Separate 1 egg into egg white and egg yolk. Throw away the egg yolk. Whip the egg white until frothy. Add egg white and mix with salmon. Set Aside. 2. Chop 2 cups red cabbage, 1 cup green pepper, 1 cup celery. 3. Add 2 cups bean sprouts. 4. Spray wok with non-aerosol oil mist. 5. Heat wok. 6. Add cabbage, green pepper and celery first. Cook. Add sprouts second. Cook. 7. Add salmon and egg mix third. Cook. 8. Add Aisan Blend spices (see Recipe).Cook. Stir-fry. 9. Serve. Makes 4 protions. Each portion equals 4 ozs protein, 1 1/2cup cooked vegetable.

• *15 ozs canned salmon • 1 egg white• 2 cups red cabbage • 1 cup green pepper• 1 cup celery • 2 cups bean sprouts. Aisan Spice Blend (see Spice Blend Recipes).*

Serving amount: 4 ozs.protein, 12 ozs. or 1 1/2 cups vegetable

Spanakopita - Spinach-Dill-Feta Pie Crustless

1. Mix all ingredients together.
2. Spray baking dish or pie plate with non-aerosol oil mist.
3. Bake at 350 degrees, 30-40 minutes.

• *8 ozs. spinach cooked and drained • dried onion flakes • 1 tbs. fresh chopped dill or dill weed or dill seed • 1 whole egg • 1 oz. crumbled feta cheese • 1 tsp. ground nutmeg*

Serving amount: 8 ozs. or 1 cup vegetable, 1 protein

Spinach-Greens-Cauliflower Creamed

1. Heat unsweetened soymilk or fat-free milkin saucepan on low.
2. Grate cheese into milk.
3. Add chopped onions to milk mixture.
4. Cook greens either in microwave or steam.
5. Add nutmeg and black pepper.
6. Chop heated greens with kitchen shears.
7. Add greens to milk-cheese-onion mixture.
8. Add 1/2 tsp. black pepper to mixture.

• *12 ozs. or 1 1/2 cup spinach or kale, brocolette or cauliflower • 1/2 cup chopped onion*
• *3/4 cup unsweetened soymilk or non-fat milk*
• *1/2 oz. cheese • 1/2 tsp. nutmeg*
• *1/2 tsp. black pepper. Makes 1 portion.*

Serving amount: 1 protein or dairy, 12 ozs.or 1 1/2 cups vegetables

Cooked Vegetables with Protein

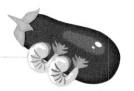

Spinach & Tomato with Garlic Chicken

1. Grill chicken breasts for 5 minutes on each side, until cooked through but not dry. Meanwhile, lightly brown the garlic in a skillet, sprayed with non-aerosol oil mist over medium-high heat.
2. Add the spinach and cook, tossing gently.
3. Add the tomatoes, soy sauce, and lemon.
4. Toss well until coated and thoroughly heated.
5. Weigh 4 ounces of chicken. Measure 1 cup of spinach and tomatoes.
6. Place spinach and tomatoes on top of cooked chicken, and serve.

• *4 boneless skinless chicken breast halves (about 2 pounds total)* • *6 cups washed loosely packed spinach (about 1 1/2 pounds)*
• *1 cup plum tomatoes* • *8-12 cloves garlic, minced* • *2 tsp. soy sauce or Bragg's amino acids (tastes like soy sauce, less sodium)* • *1 tbs. lemon*
• *non-aerosol oil mist. Makes 4 portions. Each portion equals 4 ozs. protein and 1 cup vegetable*

Serving amount: 4 ozs. protein, 1 cup vegetable

Tomato Baked with Parmesan Cheese

1. Preheat oven to 350 degrees and spray a baking pan with non-aerosol oil mist.
2. Place the tomatoes cut side up on the pan and sprinkle evenly with the black pepper, garlic powder, and then the oregano.
3. Bake until the tomatoes are tender but not squishy, approximately 8-10 minutes depending on the size and ripeness of the tomatoes.
4. Measure 8 ozs. or 1 cup tomatoes. 5. Dust with 1/2 ozs. grated parmesan cheese.

• *1/2 oz. parmesan cheese* • *2 large ripe but firm tomatoes, cut in half* • *1 tsp. oregano* • *1/4 tsp. fresh ground black pepper* • *1/2 tsp. garlic powder*
• *non-aerosol oil mist*

Serving amount: 8 ozs. or 1 cup vegetable, 1/4 protein

Cooked Vegetables with Protein

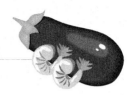

Vegetable Kabobs with Chicken - Shrimp - Lamb

1. Cut poultry & vegetables in chunks for kabobs. You may use shri mp or lamb.
2. Put kabob ingredients on skewers.
3. Brush with mustard.
4. Grill until chicken is cooked.
5. Measure vegetables and meat aftercooking.

- *4 ozs. protein: lamb cubes, beef cubes, chicken cubes, cooked, cleaned, de-veined shrimp*
- *12 ozs. or 1 1/2 cup vegetables: small tomatoes, pepper chunks, zucchini slices, eggplant cubes*
- *non-aerosol oil mist. Makes 1 portion. Each portion equals 4 ozs. protein and 1 1/2cup vegetable.*

Serving amount: 4 ozs.protein, 12 ozs. or 1 1/2 cups vegetable, non-aerosol oil mist

Cooked Vegetables with Protein with Starch/Grain

Cucumber Dill Potato Tofu Soup

1. Cook potatoes (starch) in boiling waterand measure 1/2 cup or 4 ozs.
2. Add 2 cups water and 1 cup choppedcucumbers (vegetable).
3. Heat.
4. Add tofu (dairy-free protein).
5. With a hand blender or mixer, blend allingredients in soup.

Serving amount: 1 protein, starch/grain, 1 vegetable

Peppers Stuffed with Herbed Tofu & Brown Rice

1. Preheat the oven to 350°
2. Heat a medium saucepan of water over medium heat.
3. Heat 1 tbs. oil in a large skillet over medium-high heat. Add the onion, celery, and garlic; cook until tender. Remove from heat and stir in the tofu, brown rice, tomato sauce, 2 ozs. grated Parmesan cheese, soy sauce, dried basil and oregano (if using), and pepper. When the mixture is cool to the touch, stir in the eggs and the fresh basil and oregano (if using).
4. Remove the tops and centers from the bell peppers. Stand them upright in a baking pan; if necessary, even off the bottoms so they will stand straight (avoid cutting holes). Spoon about 1/4-1/2 cup of the tofu-rice mixture into each bell pepper.

5. Pour the hot water around the peppers until about one-quarter of the way up the sides of the baking dish. Bake for about 30 to 35 minutes, or until the peppers tender when pierced with a fork. Check occasionally during the baking period and add more water to the pan if necessary.
6. Use a slotted spatula to transfer the peppers to a serving platter. Allow the peppers to stand for about 5 minutes before serving. Onion, celery tomato sauce and green peppers equals 3 cups. Tofu, parmesan cheese and eggs equals 3 proteins. Brown rice equals 3 half-cup portions. Makes 3 portions. Each portion equals 1 protein, 1 cup or 8 ozs. vegetable (or 3 peppers), and 1/2 cup starch/grain

---

- *2 tbs. olive oil*
- *1/2 cup finely chopped onion*
- *1/2 cup celery, diced*
- *1 tsp. minced garlic*
- *1/2 cup mashed silken extra-firm tofu (4 ozs.)*
- *2 large eggs, lightly beaten*
- *1 1/2 cups cooked brown rice*
- *One 8-oz. can tomato sauce*
- *2 ozs. freshly grated Parmesan cheese*
- *2 tbs. low-sodium soy sauce*
- *1 tb. minced fresh basil (or 1 tsp. dried)*
- *1 tb. minced fresh oregano (or 1 tsp. dried)*
- *1/2 tsp. freshly ground black pepper*
- *6 large green, red, or yellow bell peppers or 8 ozs. peppers*

Serving amount: 1 protein, starch/grain, 1 vegetable,1 fat daily allotment

Cooked Vegetables with Protein with Starch/Grain

Potato Salad with Hard Boiled Egg - Two-Servings

1. Cook potatoes in boiling water until soft. Rinse, drain and cool potatoes.
2. Measure 8 ozs or 1 cup portion.
3. Add chopped hardboiled eggs, choppedcelery, and chopped onion.
4. Mix together.
5. Add fat & mustard, as dressing.
6. Divide into two portions.
7. Cool in refrigerator overnight to seasonor eat directly. A food to take to picnics orfamily gatherings where others will be havingbarbeque picnic food.

- *4 ozs or 1/2 cup cooked potatoes*
- *1 hardboiled egg • 3/4 cup chopped celery*
- *1/4 cup chopped onion • 1 tb. mayonnaise*
- *1 tb. mustard*
- *1/8 tsp. dill weed• 1/8 tsp. rosemary*

Serving amount: 1 protein, starch/grain, 1 vegetable,1 fat daily allotment

Salmon Loaf or Patties With Green Pepper & Onion

1. Open large can of canned salmon.
2. Chop 1 cup green pepper & 1 cup onion.
3. Mix 1 cup raw oatbran or raw oatmeal with 1 egg, chopped green pepper and choppedonion.
4. Mix all ingredients well until well blended.
5. Put salmon loaf ingredients into large loaf pan.
6. Bake salmon loaf for 20-30 minutes at 325 degrees.
7. Cut salmon loaf into 4 portions. Makes 4 portions. Each portion equals 4 ozs. protein, 1 oz. dry or 1/2 cup cooked starch/grain, 1/2 cup vegetable.

- *15 ozs. can canned salmon. • 1 raw egg*
- *4 ozs. dry oat bran or dry oatmeal*
- *1 cup green pepper • 1 cup onion.*

Serving amount: 4 ozs. protein, 1 oz. dry or1/2 cup cooked starch/grain.

Raw Vegetables

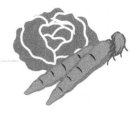

3 Raws Dip

1. Process all ingredients in food processor.
2. Microwave to melt cheese and meld flavors (couple minutes on high usually).
3. Dip your 3 raws to your heart's content.

• *3 ozs. canned soybeans* • *1 oz. soycheese (any kind, pepperjack/cheddar combo)* • *onion powder* • *garlic powder* • *celery seed powder* • *hot pepper flakes* • *4 ozs. rotel tomatoes (these are canned tomatoes w/green chili peppers)* • *include some of the juice when you measure to make the dip spread smoother* • *1/2 tsp. salt (or to taste)* • *4 oz canned mushrooms*

Serving amount: 3 raw vegetables or 1 1/2 cups vegetable

3 Raws Salad

1. Mix and enjoy!

• *4 ozs. yogurt* • *2 ozs. soy nuts (mix in at end right before eating)* • *3 raw vegetables* • *allowable portion of oil for meal (sesame oil toasted is best)* • *brown mustard* • *vinegar*

Serving amount: 4 ozs. or 1/2 cup dairy, 2 ozs. protein, 3 raw vegetables or 1 1/2 cup vegetable

Cabbage and Carrot Cole Slaw

1. Measure cabbage and carrots into one bowl.
2. Add allowable portion of mayonnaise and vinegar and mix together.
3. Prepare a few minutes early, and let the mixture sit, to fully marry the flavors together.
4. Restir and serve.
5. For a sweeter cole slaw, add more sweetener.

• *1 1/2 cups shredded cabbage and 1/2 cup carrots* • *1/2 tbs. vinegar* • *salt and pepper, or abstinent seasoned salt* • *sweetener (optional)*

Serving amount: 4 ozs. or 1/2 cup starchy vegetable, 1 1/2 cup vegetable

Cabbage and Pepper Fiesta Slaw

1. Slice red and white cabbage in a food processor, or grater, or by hand, in long thin strips.
2. Dice red, green, and yellow bell peppers into small cubes.
3. Toss together.
4. After measuring one serving, measure your oil allowance, and add on top.
5. You may also add a few drops of lemon juice.

• *red cabbage* • *white cabbage* • *red bell pepper* • *green bell pepper* • *yellow bell pepper*

Serving amount: 1 1/2 cup vegetable

Raw Vegetables

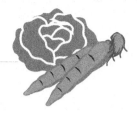

Carrot, Shredded Carrot Salad

1. Peel carrots and either food process or grate by hand to make a shredded slaw consistency.
2. Mix in mayo, sweetener to taste, and just a dash of salt.
3. Refrigerate

- *3 raw carrots • 1 tsp. mayonnaise*
- *sweetener (optional)*

Serving amount: 3 raw vegetables or 1/2 cup starchy vegetable, 1 tsp. oil

Cauliflower Slaw With Creamy Dill Dressing

1. Trim the cauliflower and cut it into small florets. Steam the florets until they lose their raw taste but are still firm and crunchy, 3 to 4 minutes. Run under cold water to stop cook¬ing, then drain thoroughly.
2. Place the florets in the bowl of a food processor and use the pulsing action to chop them coarsely.
3. Transfer to a serving bowl. Toss in the bell pepper, onion, and enough dressing to thoroughly coat the mixture. Adjust the seasonings with salt, pepper, and the lemon juice (if using).

- *1 medium head (about 2 pounds) cauliflower*
- *1 large red bell pepper, roasted, peeled, seeded, and finely diced • 1/2 cup minced red onion*
- *1/2 to 2/3 cup creamy dill dressing salt and freshly ground black pepper to taste, freshly squeezed lemon juice to taste (optional).*

Serving amount: 12 ozs. or 1 1/2 cup vegetable

Cole Slaw I

1. Shred cabbage finely.
2. Crisp cabbage in cold water for an hour.
3. Drain well.
4. Measure portion for salad serving.
5. Add allowable portion of oil and seasonings.
6. Toss well and let stand for 30 minutes or longer.
7. Serve cold.

- *1 head cabbage • allowable portion of oil*
- *1 tsp. dijon mustard • salt • pepper*

Serving amount: 12 ozs. or 1 1/2 cup vegetables

Cole Slaw II - No Mayo

1. Mix together cabbage and seasonings.

- *1 package pre-shredded cabbage • sweetener (optional) • salt to taste • 1/4 tsp. vinegar (or to taste) • 1 tsp. dill seed or weed*

Serving amount: 12 ozs. or 1 1/2 cup vegetables

Raw Vegetables

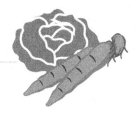

Cole Slaw III - Fiesta Slaw

1. Slice red and white cabbage in a food processer or grater or by hand in long thin strips.
2. Dice red and green and yellow bell pepper into small cubes.
3. Toss together.
4. Measure 1 cup or 8 ozs.
5. Toss Fiesta Slaw. Use non-aerosol oil mist.

• *red cabbage* • *white cabbage* • *red bell pepper* • *green bell pepper* • *yellow bell pepper*

Serving amount: 12 ozs. or 1 1/2 cup vegetables, non-aerosol oil mist

Cole Slaw IV - Festiva with Tofu Croutons

1. In a large serving bowl or storage container, combine the cabbage, bell pepper, scallions, and diced tofu.
2. Toss in enough dressing to coat the slaw thoroughly.

• *1 pound napa cabbage, shredded (5 to 6 cups)* • *1 cup finely diced red bell pepper* • *1/2 cup thinly sliced scallion greens* • *4 ozs. baked seasoned tofu , cut into 1/4-inch dice (about 1 cup)* • *dressing and dipping sauce of choice.*

Serving amount: 12 ozs. or 1 1/2 cup vegetable, non-aerosol oil mist

Cucumber Salad - Asian Taste

1. Mix all ingredients in a bowl. 2. Weigh, measure and enjoy.

• *2 cucumbers* • *soy sauce* • *fresh mint* • *lime juice* • *chili garlic sauce (from Asian food market, jar has a green lid and a rooster on the front (ingredients: chili, vinegar, garlic, salt, potassium sorbate and sodium bisulfite).*

Serving amount: 12 ozs. or 1 1/2 cup vegetables

Cucumbers - Dill

1. Save juice from dill pickles.
2. Put cucumbers in jar with juice.
3. Measure for raw veggies.

• *dill pickle juice (no sugar)* • *3 cucumbers.*

Serving amount: 12 ozs. or 1 1/2 cup vegetables

Cucumbers - Sweet

1. Mix vinegar, dill and sweetener (optional) together.
2. Pour mixture over cucumbers.
3. Chill and add these to salad.

• *1 cup sliced cucumbers* • *1 tsp. white vinegar or lemon juice* • *sweetener (optional)*

Serving amount: 12 ozs. or 1 1/2 cup

Raw Vegetables

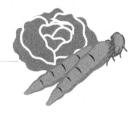

Gaspacho I - Cold Vegetable Soup

1. Combine all ingredients. Blend slightly, to desired consistency.
2. Place in a non-metal storage container, cover tightly and refrigerate overnight, allowing flavors to blend.
3. Measure portion to be used.

• *6 ripe tomatoes, peeled and shopped*
• *1 purple onion* • *1 cucumber, peeled and chopped* • *1 sweet red pepper or green, chopped*
• *2 stalks celery, chopped* • *1 tbs. fresh parsley, chopped* • *1 clove garlic* • *4 cups tomato juice (no sugar)* • *6 drops Tabasco sauce or 1 tsp. cayanne pepper* • *2 tbs lemon juice* • *1/8 cup vinegar*
• *1/2 tsp.salt* • *1/2 tsp. pepper*

Serving amount: 12 ozs. or 1 1/2 cup

Gaspacho II - Cold Vegetable Soup with Lime & Jalapeno

1. Combine all ingredients. Blend slightly, to desired consistency.
2. Place in a non-metal storage container, cover tightly and refrigerate overnight, allowing flavors to blend.
3. Measure portion to be used.

• *6 ripe tomatoes, peeled and shopped*
• *1 purple onion* • *1 cucumber, peeled and chopped* • *1 sweet red pepper or green, chopped*
• *1 tbs. fresh parsley, chopped* • *1 clove garlic*
• *4 cups tomato juice (no sugar)*
• *1 small jalapeno chili, chopped and minced*
• *2 tbs. lime juice* • *1/8 cup vinegar*
• *1/2 tsp.salt* • *1/2 tsp. pepper*

Serving amount: 12 ozs. or 1 1/2 cup

Vegetables Pickled, Claussen Crunch

1. Mix the raw cauliflower, tomatoes, dillpickles, onion and dill weed in a large bowl,then transferred it to a gallon zip-lock bag.
2. Measured out 8 ounces of this mixture.
3. Add 1 tbs. lemon or vinegar and 1 tsp. oil.
4. Let this mixture set overnight in a coveredcontainer in the fridge.
5. Mix well.

• *1 head raw cauliflower rinsed, trimmed, cut in bite-size pieces* • *15-20 cherry tomatoes cut in1/4ths (or 2 large tomatoes, chopped)*
• *4-5 dill pickle spears cut in 1/2" slices (no sugar)* • *1/2 small onion peeled & chopped*
• *1 tsp. dill weed* • *1 tb. lemon juice or vinegar*
• *non-aerosol oil mist*

Serving amount: 12 ozs. or 1 1/2 cup

Zucchini Summer Squash Salad

1. Dice up all 3 raw vegetables.
2. Toss with oil, vinegar and rosemary orbasil.

• *3 zucchini* • *1 tsp. basil* • *1 tsp. dill weed or seed or rosemary* • *1 tb. lemon juice or vinegar*
• *non-aerosol oil mist*

Serving amount: 12 ozs. or 1 1/2 cup vegetable, non-aerosol oil mist

Raw Vegetables With Protein

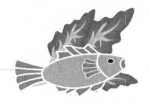

Broccoli Salad

1. Cook bacon and cut into small pieces.
2. Mix together broccoli and bacon.
3. Add 1 tsp. no-sugar mayonnaise or oil.

• *1 cup chopped raw broccoli (may use choppedbroccoli from store)* • *1/2 cup chopped celery* • *1 oz. cooked bacon cut into small pieces* • *1 tsp. oil or mayonnaise*

Serving amount: 1 ozs. protein, 12 ozs. or 11/2 cup vegetable. 1 tsp. oil

Caprese Little Salads - Mozarella-Tomato-Basil With Olive Oil

1. Slice fresh tomato - 8 ozs.into medium sizeround slices.
2. Slice mozzarella cheese - 2 oz. into thin round slices.
3. Break sprigs of fresh basil with leaves onlyinto small spoon size portions.
4. Measure 2 tsp. olive oil into small bowl with pour lip.
5. Build "capreses" (an Italian small salad) by taking a slice of tomato, putting mozzarellaslices on top of tomato, and basil leaves ontop, and sprinkling with small amounts of measured olive oil. Or spray with oil mist.

• *1 cup or 8 ozs fresh tomato slices* • *2 ozs slicedmozzarella cheese* • *1 ozs. fresh basil leaves* • *2 tsp.olive oil*

Serving amount: 2 ozs cheese for 1complete portion protein, 8 ozs. or 1 cup vegetable, 2 tsp. oil

Club Salad - Chicken, Bacon, Lettuce

1. Stir allowable portion of dressing for thismeal into chicken.
2. Place lettuce leaves onplate.
3. Add tomatoes.
4. Add chicken. 5.Top with bacon.

• *3 1/2 ozs. chicken* • *1/2 oz. bacon*
• *1 cup lettuce* • *1/2 cup diced tomatoes.*

Serving amount: 4 ozs. protein, 12 ozs. or 1 1/2 cup vegetable

Crab Louis Salad

1. Mix crab, tomato sauce, and allowable portion of oil or mayonnaise together.
2. Serve on top of 1 1/2 cups lettuce.
3. This is best made with Dungeness crab, but lump crabmeat is almost as good.
4. Meat from lobster tails may also be used. Variation: 1/4 cup crab and 1 hard-boiled egg, sliced.

• *1/2 cup crab* • *1 1/2 cups shredded lettuce*
• *2 ozs. tomato sauce or chili sauce*
• *1 tbs. mock sour cream.*

Serving amount: 4 ozs. protein, 12 ozs. or 1 1/2 cup vegetable, non-aerosol oil mist

Raw Vegetables With Protein

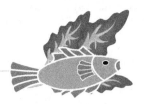

Crab Salad

1. Mix greens, celery, and onion.
2. Stir in mustard and allowable portion of mayonnaise.
3. Chill for 2 to 3 hours.
4. Top with crabmeat and serve.

• *1/2 cup crabmeat* • *1 1/4 cup lettuce greens* • *1/4 cup finely cut celery* • *1/4 cup finely cut onion* • *mustard* • *allowable portion of oil or mayonnaise*

Serving amount: 4 ozs. protein, 12 ozs. or 1 1/2 cup vegetable, non-aerosol oil mist

Cucumbers and Cream

1. Whip cottage cheese, herbs, and salt to taste, in blender.
2. Spread on cucumbers.

• *1/2 cup cottage cheese* • *3 raw, sliced cucumbers* • *2 tsp. of fresh herbs (dill or chives)* • *salt*

Serving amount: 4 ozs. protein, 12 ozs. or 1 1/2 cup vegetable, non-aerosol oil mist

Ham Salad with Celery & Onions

1. Combine ham, celery, green onions, and chopped pickles.
2. Bind with allowable portion of mayonnaise and mustard.
3. Arrange on greens and top with tomatoes.

• *4 ozs. diced cold ham* • *1/2 cup lettuce greens* • *1/2 cup finely chopped celery* • *1/2 cup finely cut green onions* • *1/4 cup chopped tomatoes* • *1/4 cup finely chopped pickles* • *mayonnaise* • *mustard*

Serving amount: 4 ozs. protein, 12 ozs. or 1 1/2 cup vegetable, non-aerosol oil mist

Mesclun with Brie, Sun-Dried Tomatoes, Smoked Turkey

1. Wash fresh mesclun leaves. Measure 4 ozs. weighed mesclum leaves.
2. Chop 1 ozs. sun-dried tomatoes and 1 oz. brie cheese and 2 ozs. smoked turkey and put in salad.
3. Put sun-dried tomatoes, briw cheese and smoked turkey on top of salad.
4. Toss salad.
5. Spray salad with non-aerosol oil mist. Or use Mustard Dill Dressing or Spice Blends.

• *11 ozs. mesclum leaves* • *1 oz. sun-dried tomatoes* • *1 oz. brie cheese* • *2 ozs. smoked turkey* • *non-aerosol oil mist*

Serving amount: 4 ozs. protein, 12 ozs. or 1 1/2 cup vegetable, non-aerosol oil mist

Raw Vegetables With Protein

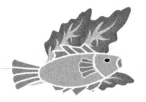

Romaine Lettuce with Fresh Tomato, Cucumber & Grilled Chicken

1. Wash fresh romaine lettuce leaves. Measure 4 ozs. romaine leaves.
2. Chop fresh tomato to make 4 ozs., chop cucumber to make 4 ozs., and chop grilled chicken to make 4 ozs.
3. Toss salad.
4. Spray salad with non-aerosol oil mist.

- *4 ozs. romaine lettuce* • *4 ozs. chopped tomato*
- *4 ozs. chopped cucumbers* • *4 ozs. chopped grilled chicken* • *non-aerosol oil mist*

Serving amount: 4 ozs. protein, 12 ozs. or 1 1/2 cup vegetable, non-aerosol oil mist

Salad, Chef's Style

1. Measure out salad vegetables.
2. Add weighed cold cuts, such as ham, turkey, chicken, salami, or soy cold cuts.
3. Top with weighed shredded cheese, such as cheddar, american, or mozarella.
4. Add allowable portion of salad dressing.
5. Sprinkle on favorite abstinent salad spices. Make sure that cold cuts and dressing have sugar as fifth, or lower, ingredient.

- *1 1/2 cups salad* • *2 ozs. cold cuts*
- *1 oz. shredded cheese* • *non-aerosol oil mist*

Serving amount: 4 ozs. protein, 12 ozs. or 1 1/2 cup vegetable, non-aerosol oil mist

Salad, Taco Style

1. Measure out taco-style salad vegetables, such as lettuce, tomato, carrots, etc.
2. Stir cooked ground beef or soy in with cooked onions and tomato sauce.
3. Top salad with cooked meat and onions.
4. Add allowable portion of ranch dressing on top.

- *8 ozs. or 1 cup salad* • *4 ozs. cooked ground beef*
- *1/2 cup sauteed onions* • *2 ozs. tomato sauce, taco spices* • *non-aerosol oil mist.*

Serving amount: 4 ozs. protein, 12 ozs. or 1 1/2 cup vegetable, non-aerosol oil mist

Salmon Salad

1. Combine flaked salmon with vegetables.
2. Toss well with allowable portion of mayonnaise. Variation: Use spinach as the greens.

- *1/2 cup flaked cold poached salmon*
- *1/2 cup greens* • *1/2 cup sliced, peeled, and seeded cucumber* • *1/2 cup finely cut celery*
- *1/2 cup finely cut green onions* • *mayonnaise*

Serving amount: 4 ozs. protein, 12 ozs. or 1 1/2 cup vegetable, non-aerosol oil mist

Raw Vegetables With Protein

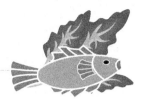

Spinach Leaves with Blue Cheese & Cucumber

1. Wash fresh spinach leaves. Measure 4 ozs. weighed spinach leaves. 2. Chop 1 hard boiled egg and 1 oz. blue cheese and put in salad. 3. Chop 1 fresh cucumber and measure 1 cup or 8 ozs. Put cucumber in salad. 4. Toss salad. 5. Spray salad with non-aerosol oil mist.

- *4 ozs. spinach leaves • 1 hard boiled egg*
- *1 ozs. blue cheese • 8 ozs. or 1 cup cucumber*
- *non-aerosol oil mist*

Serving amount: 4 ozs. protein, 12 ozs. or 1 1/2 cup vegetable, non-aerosol oil mist

Fats - Oils - Dressing - Sauces

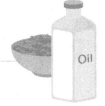

Barbecue Sauce

1. Mix well.
2. Store in a container in fridge.

___

- *1/2 cup un-ketchup (see recipe)*
- *1 tbs. soysauce.* • *a dash or 2 of tobasco sauce (no sugar), sweetener (optional)*
- *or Barbeque Spice Blend (See Barbeque Spice Blend Recipe).*

Cole Slaw Dressing I

1. Mix ingredients.
2. Measure 1 tbs. dressing for each 2 cups cole slaw.
3. Mix with shredded cabbage and carrots.
4. Toss.

___

- *1 oz. mayonnaise* • *1 oz. mustard*
- *1/2 oz. sesame oil or peanut oil*
- *1/2 oz. apple cider vinegar*

Serving amount:1 tsp.-1 tbs. fat-oil (measured)

Blue Cheese Dressing

1. Take sour cream, whole milk and blue cheese and mix together.

___

- *3 tbs. mock sour cream* • *1/4 cup whole milk*
- *1.375 oz. blue cheese*

Serving amount:1 tsp.-1 tbs. fat-oil (measured)

Cole Slaw Dressing II

1. Mix all ingredients together in a jar.
2. Close lid tightly.
3. Shake vigorously.
4. Keep refrigerated and measure outportion of fat before using.

___

- *1 1/2 cup oil* • *3 tsp. onion flakes*
- *1/2 cup vinegar* • *1 tsp. celery seed*
- *1 pint real mayonnaise*
- *3 tbs. chopped dill no sugar pickle* • *sweetener (optional)*

Serving amount:1 tsp.-1 tbs. fat-oil (measured)

Fats - Oils - Dressing - Sauces

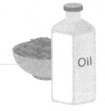

Dill Tofu Creamy Dressing

1. Put the tofu in a fine-mesh strainer and set aside to drain for 15 minutes.
2. With the motor of the food processor running, pop the garlic through the feed tube. Process until finely chopped. Remove the cover, scrape down the sides of the work bowl, and add the drained tofu and the remaining ingredients. Process until smooth, stopping and scraping down the work bowl once or twice as needed.
3. Use immediately or transfer to a tightly sealed storage container and refrigerate for up to 3 days. Makes 8 portions. Each portion equals 1 oz. protein, 1/2 tbs. oil

---

- *1 cup (8 ozs.) silken soft tofu*
- *1 small clove garlic, peeled*
- *l cup tightly packed fresh dill (stems removed)*
- *1/4 cup freshly squeezed lemon juice*
- *4 tbs. olive oil • 1 tb. dijon mustard • 1 tsp. salt*

Serving amount:1 oz. protein, 1 tbs oil

Ketchup Homemade (No Sugar)

1. Add all ingredients.
2. Cover.
3. Microwave on high for 2 minutes untilthick.
4. Allow to cool. 5. Keep refrigerated. 6. Measure allotted amount.

- *1 small can tomato paste • 2 small cans tomato sauce • 1/4 cup vinegar • 1/2 tsp. celery powder • 2 tbs. dehydrated onion flakes • 2 tsp. onion powder • 1 tb. cinnamon powder • 2 tsp. salt • 8 whole cloves • 1/4 tsp. chili*

Serving amount:1 tsp.-1 tbs. fat-oil (measured)

Lime Shoyu Tofu Vinaigrette Dressing

1 Put all the ingredients in a small jar and shake well.
2. Use immedi¬ately or refrigerate for up to 5 days.
3. Bring to room temperature and shake well before using.

- *1/3 cup freshly squeezed lime juice*
- *1/4 cup olive oil • 2 tbs. shoyu*
- *2 tsp. dijon mustard*

Serving amount:1 tsp.-1 tbs. fat-oil

Fats - Oils - Dressing - Sauces

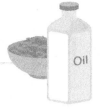

Mayonnaise-Salsa Salad Dressing

1. Mix all ingredients together in a jar.
2. Close lid tightly.
3. Shake vigorously.
4. Keep refrigerated and measure portion of dressing as fat before using. Makes (3) portions. Each portion equals 1 tbs. fat.

• *3 tbs. mayonnaise* • *2 oz. salsa*
• *add mustard, to taste.*

Serving amount:1 tsp.-1 tbs. fat-oil (measured)

Mock Sour Cream I

1. In a blender combine the ingredients.
2. Blend on pulse a few times only.
3. Store mock sour cream in airtight container. Use within 2 days. Makes 1 portions. Each portion equals 1/3 dairy, 1/2 protein.

• *1/3 cup yogurt* • *1/4 cup cottage cheese*
• *1 tsp. vinegar*

Serving amount:1/3 dairy, 1/2 protein

Mock Sour Cream II

1. Pulse tofu and vinegar in a blender.
2. Refrigerate for up to 4 days. Makes about 4 portions. Each portion equals 1 ozs. protein.

• *4 ozs. silken tofu* • *1 tsp. vinegar.*

Oil & Vinegar Dressing

1. Combine all ingredients in a jar.
2. Close lid tightly.
3. Shake vigorously.
4. Measure allotted amount.
Keep refrigerated and measure ou tportion of fat each time before using.

• *3/4 cup olive oil* • *1/4 cup vinegar* • *1 shallot, finely chopped or 1/4 cup onion* • *1/4 tsp. salt* • *1/4 tsp. freshly ground pepper*

Serving amount: 1 tsp.-1 tbs. fat-oil

Fats - Oils - Dressing - Sauces

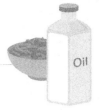

Soynut or Soynut Butter - Lime - Ginger Dressing

1. Peel the gingerroot.
2. Put all of the ingredients in a blender.
3. Process until the gineger root is finely chopped and the soynuts are slightly chunky or the soynut butter blended.
4. Use as a dressing on salads or vegetables. Makes 4 portions. Each portion equals 1/4 protein, 1/4 fruit.

• *1/2 cup dry roasted soynuts or 2 ozs. soynut butter* • *1 piece ginger root about 2 inches long x 1 inch thick, peeled* • *1 tsp. red hot chili pepper or to taste* • *1/4 cup fresly squeezed lime juice or juice of 2 limes* • *2 tbs. soy suace or Bragg's amino acids (tastes like soy only less sodium)*

Serving amount: 1/4 protein, 1/4 fruit

Soynut Butter-Miso Dressing & Dipping Sauce

1. With a food processor or blender, pop the garlic and then the ginger through the feed tube and continue to process until they are finely chopped. Remove the lid, scrape down the work bowl, and add 1/3 cup of water, the soynut butter, miso, and shoyu. Blend until smooth.
2. Add the lime juice and a dash of chili oil (if using), and pulse a few times to distribute. Thin with additional water, if you wish. Use immediately or refrigerate for up to 3 days. Shake well before each use and thin with extra lime juice or water if the mixture thickens on standing. Makes 4 portions. Each portion equals 1/2 oz. soynut butter or 1/4 protein.

• *1 large clove garlic, peeled*
• *2-inch chunk fresh ginger, trimmed and cut into eighths* • *1/3 to 1/2 cup hot water*
• *2 ozs. soynut butter butter*
• *2 tbs. sweet white miso*
• *1 tb. shoyu or Bragg's amino acids (tastes like soy sauce with less sodium)*
• *3 tbs. freshly squeezed lime juice* •
 chili oil or ground cayenne pepper, to taste (optional)

Serving amount: 1/2 oz. soynut butter or 1/4 protein

Fats - Oils - Dressing - Sauces

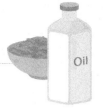

Tofu Caesar Salad Dressing

1. Pulse cheese and garlic in a blender.
2. Add vinegar and mustard and blend.
3. Add tofu, oil, salt and pepper, blend.
4. Refrigerate for up to 1 week. Makes about 1 portion. Each portion equals 1 tsp. oil, 4 ozs. protein.

- *3 ozs. silken tofu • 1 tsp. vinegar*
- *1 tsp. dry mustard • 1 clove garlic crushed*
- *1 oz. grated parmesan cheese • 1 tb. olive oil*
- *1/4 tsp. each salt and coarse black pepper.*

Serving amount:1 tsp. oil, 4 ozs. protein

Tofu Cucumber Dill Dressing

1. Cut cucumber into chunks.
2. Combine ingredients and place in a blender. Blend.
3. Refrigerate in an airtight container for up to 1 week. Makes 1 portion. Each portion equals 1/2 cup or 4 ozs. raw vegetable and 4 ozs. protein.

- *4 ozs. silken tofu • 1 tsp. vinegar*
- *4 ozs. or 1/2 cup fresh cucumber*
- *1/8 cup fresh dill weed or 1 tb. chopped dill weed and dill seed • 1/8 cup vinegar*
- *1/4 tsp. each salt and coarse black pepper*

Serving amount: 4 ozs. or 1/2 cup vegetable, 4 ozs. protein, 1/2 tbs. oil

Tofu Mayonnaise

1. Blend all ingredients in a blender.
2. Keep refrigerated in an airtight container up to 1 week. Makes about 1/2 cup. Makes 2 servings. Each 1/4 cup serving equals 1/2 tbs. oil and 2 ozs. tofu or 1/2 protein.

- *4 ozs. firm tofu • 1 tb. oil • 1/2 tsp. dry mustard • 1/2 tsp. no alcohol lemon extract. add salt, to taste.*

Serving amount:1/2 tbs. oil, 2 ozs. tofu or 1/2 protein

Yogurt - Mustard Dip for Steamed Broccoli

1. Mix 1/2 cup yogurt with mustard and vinegar.

- *1/2 cup yogurt • 1 tb. mustard • 1 tsp. vinegar*

Serving amount: 4 ozs. dairy or protein

Seasonings - Spice Blends - Condiments

Making Spice Blends

1. Using herbs is a delicious way to season dishes and cut the amount of salt needed for flavor. Fresh herbs need to be used immediately. Dried herb mixtures can be prepared in advance and stored in an airtight container.
2. To prepare fresh herbs, dry them by putting them on a baking sheet and bake at 200 degrees for 30 minutes.
3. Blends can be made from whole seeds or leaves by coarsley grinding them in a spice grinder to by a hand blender or in a food processor.
4. Basically, nuts, seeds, and roots are spices; leafy plants are herbs.

Barbeque Blend

• *4 tbs. dried basil* • *3 tsp. cracked black pepper*
• *4 tbs. dried rubbed sage* • *4 tbs. dried thyme* • *4 tsp. dried savory* • *1 tsp. dried lemon peel*

Serving amount: Not counted toward a nutritional food group serving. To flavor, 1tsp. - 1 tbs. blend to taste.

Cajun Blend

• *1 tsp. cayenne pepper* • *2 tsp. dried oregano*
• *2 tbs. paprika* • *1 1/2 tbs. garlic powder*
• *1 tbs. onion powder* • *1/2 tbs. black pepper*
• *2 tsp. dried thyme*

Serving amount: Not counted toward a nutritional food group serving. To flavor, 1tsp. - 1 tbs. blend to taste.

Caribbean Blend

• *1 tbs. ground cumin* • *1 tbs. ground allspice*
• *1/2 tbs. curry powder* • *1 tbs. ground ginger*
• *1 tsp. ground cayenne pepper*

Serving amount: Not counted toward a nutritional food group serving. To flavor, 1tsp. - 1 tbs. blend to taste.

Country Blend

• *4 tsp. dried tarragon* • *4 tsp. dried thyme*
• *4 tsp. dried basil* • *4 tsp. dried chervil*

Serving amount: Not counted toward a nutritional food group serving. To flavor, 1tsp. - 1 tbs. blend to taste.

Fish and Seafood Herbs

• *4 tsp. crushed fennel seed* • *4 tsp. dried basil*
• *4 tsp. dried parsley* • *1 tsp. dried lemon peel*

Serving amount: Not counted toward a nutritional food group serving. To flavor, 1tsp. - 1 tbs. blend to taste.

French Blend

• *1 tbs. crushed dried tarragon*
• *1 tbs. crushed dried chervil*
• *1 tbs. onion powder*

Serving amount: Not counted toward a nutritional food group serving. To flavor, 1tsp. - 1 tbs. blend to taste.

Seasonings - Spice Blends - Condiments

Herbes de Provence

- *3 tsp. dried oregano* • *1 tsp. dried basil*
- *1 tsp. dried sweet marjoram* • *1 tsp. dried thyme* • *1 tsp. dried mint* • *1 tsp. dried rosemary*
- *1 tsp. dried sage leaves* • *1 tsp. fennel seed* • *1 tsp. dried lavender (optional)*

Serving amount: Not counted toward a nutritional food group serving. To flavor, 1tsp. - 1 tbs. blend to taste.

Italian Blend

- *1 tbs. crushed dried basil* • *1 tbs. crushed dried thyme* • *1 tbs. crushed dried oregano*
- *2 tbs. garlic powder* • *2 tsp. fennel seeds*

Serving amount: Not counted toward a nutritional food group serving. To flavor, 1tsp. - 1 tbs. blend to taste.

Lemon & Garlic Blend

- *2 tbs. lemon juice* • *1 tbs. fresh minced garlic or 1 tbs. minced garlic from a jar or 1 tbs. garlicpowder. Rub on fish and meat.*

Serving amount: Not counted toward a nutritional food group serving. To flavor, 1tsp. - 1 tbs. blend to taste.

Mediterranean Blend

- *1 tbs. dried sun-dried tomatoes* • *1 tbs. dried basil*
- *1 tsp. dried oregano* • *1 tsp. dried thyme*
- *1 tbs. garlic powder*

Serving amount: Not counted toward a nutritional food group serving. To flavor, 1tsp. - 1 tbs. blend to taste.

Middle Eastern Blend

- *1 tbs. ground coriander* • *1 tbs. ground cumin*
- *1 tbs. turmeric* • *1 tsp. ground cinnamon*
- *1 tsp. crushed dried mint* • *2 tbs. parsley*

Serving amount: Not counted toward a nutritional food group serving. To flavor, 1tsp. - 1 tbs. blend to taste.

Old Bay Seasoning

- *1 tbs. celery seed* • *1 tbs. whole black peppercorns*
- *3 bay leaves* • *1/2 tsp. whole cardamom*
- *1/2 tsp. mustard seed* • *2 whole cloves*
- *1 tsp. sweet Hungarian paprika* • *1/4 tsp. mace*

Serving amount: Not counted toward a nutritional food group serving. To flavor, 1tsp. - 1 tbs. blend to taste.

Seasonings - Spice Blends - Condiments

Pacific Rim Blend

- *1 tbs. Chinese five-spice powder • 1 tbs. paprika*
- *1 tbs. ground ginger • 1 tsp. black pepper.*

Serving amount: Not counted toward a nutritional food group serving. To flavor, 1tsp. - 1 tbs. blend to taste.

Sonoran Mexico Blend

- *1 tbs. ground chili powder • 1 tbs. black pepper*
- *1 tbs. crushed dried oregano • 1 tbs. crushed dried thyme • 1 tbs. crushed driedcoriander*
- *1 tbs. garlic powder*

Serving amount: Not counted toward a nutritional food group serving. To flavor, 1tsp. - 1 tbs. blend to taste.

Swedish Spice Blend

- *1 tbs. ground cardamon • 1 tbs. ground nutmeg*
- *1 tbs. ground cinnamon*

Serving amount: Not counted toward a nutritional food group serving. To flavor, 1tsp. - 1 tbs. blend to taste.

Texas Seasoning Blend

- *3 tbs. dried cilantro • 2 tbs. dried oregano • 4 tsp. dried thyme • 2 tbs. pure good-quality chili powder*
- *2 tbs. freshly ground black pepper• 2 tbs. ground cumin • 2 small crushed driedchili peppers • 1 tsp. garlic powder*

Serving amount: Not counted toward a nutritional food group serving. To flavor, 1tsp. - 1 tbs. blend to taste.

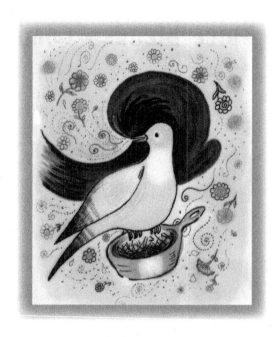

CHAPTER 9

People and Groups

FREE PHONE MEETINGS
ONLINE & FACE-TO-FACE MEETINGS
SPONSOR & PHONE BUDDY CONTACTS
PHONE NUMBERS - WEBSITES - EMAILS
PLANS OF EATING SUPPORTED
WEIGHING & MEASURING PRACTICES

CEA-HOW (Compulsive Overeaters Anonymous-HOW)

http://www.ceahow.org/
5500 E. Atherton St., Suite 227-B
Long Beach, CA 90815-4017
562-342-9344
CEA-HOW General Service Office: gso@ceahow

- "Compulsive Eaters Anonymous-HOW is a fellowship of individuals who, through shared experience, strength, and hope are recovering from compulsive eating and food addiction. We welcome everyone who wants to stop eating compulsively. There are no dues or fees for members; we are self-supporting through our own contributions, neither soliciting nor accepting outside donations. CEA-HOW is not affiliated with any public or private organization, political movement, ideology, or religious doctrine; we take no position on outside issues. Our primary purpose is to abstain from compulsive eating and to carry the message of recovery to those who still suffer. The Compulsive Eaters Anonymous-HOW Concept has been formed to offer the compulsive eater who accepts the Twelve Steps and Twelve Traditions as a program of recovery a disciplined and structured approach.

  The CEA-HOW Groups have been formed in the belief that our disease is absolute and therefore only absolute acceptance of the CEA-HOW Concept will offer any sustained abstinence to those of us whose compulsion has reached a critical level. Therefore, the CEA-HOW plan of eating, steps, traditions and tools of recovery are not suggested. Rather, we accept them as requirements for our recovery (http://www.ceahow.org). Note: CEA-HOW is not affiliated with Overeaters Anonymous or the OA-HOW meetings, where refraining from sugar and flour or following a specific plan of eating is a suggestion and not a requirement" (CEA-HOW Website, http://www.ceahow.org, May 2010).

  There is a required plan of eating. It includes fruit, dairy, protein and vegetables. The CEA-HOW plan of eating is available from "Achieving Balance Cookbook" at the website:
  http://www.ceahow.org/?q=node/11

Are there phone meetings?
- Yes

How do I get a list of phone meetings?
- To Get Started: Phone Meetings Daily: 5:30 a.m., 7 a.m., 10 a.m., 1 p.m.,4 p.m., 5 p.m., 7 p.m., 6:45 p.m., 9 p.m., 10:30 p.m., 11 p.m., 12 Midnight, EST. • Figure the meeting time at your time zone. • Phone Number: (712)-432-1680, access code: 152077#.
- Go to: http://www.ceahow-org?g=content/phone-bridge-meetings for a complete list of phone meetings

- How do I get a list of "We Care" phone numbers & email addresses, people willing to help?
- Click on: http://tinyurl.com/24kzgos for Phone Numbers & Email addresses for Phone Buddies, Action Partners & Sponsors, and to volunteer to be a Phone Buddy, Action Partner or Sponsor.
- Send an email to: phonebridgeoutreach@gmail.com for a list of Phone Numbers, Email addresses for Phone Buddies, Action Partners & Sponsors, and to volunteer to be a Phone Buddy, Action Partner or Sponsor.

What are the types of phone meetings?
- 12 & 12
- AA Big Book
- AA Comes of Age
- As Bill Sees It
- Came to Believe
- Daily Reflections
- Living Sober
- Promises
- Relapse Prevention
- Speaker Qualification
- Steps/Traditions
- The CEA-HOW Concept
- Topic Discussion

Are there all day phone marathons?
- No

Are there online meetings?
- No

Are there face-to-face meetings?
- Yes

How do I get a list of face-to-face meetings?
- Click on: http://tinyurl.com/27aoofu for a list of Face-to-Face Meetings.

What are the types of face-to-face meetings?
- 12 & 12
- AA Big Book
- AA Comes of Age
- As Bill Sees It
- Came to Believe
- Daily Reflections
- Living Sober
- Promises
- Relapse Prevention
- Speaker Qualification
- Steps/Traditions
- The CEA-HOW Concept
- Topic Discussion

Are there sponsors, phone buddies & action partners?
- Yes

How do I get a sponsor, phone buddy or action partner?
How do I get a list of "We Care" phone numbers & email addresses, people available for outreach
- Click on: http://tinyurl.com/24kzgos for Phone Numbers & Email addresses for Phone Buddies, Action Partners & Sponsors, and to volunteer to be a Phone Buddy, Action Partner or Sponsor.
- Send an email to: phonebridgeoutreach@gmail.com for a list of Phone Numbers, Email addresses for Phone Buddies, Action Partners & Sponsors, and to volunteer to be a Phone Buddy, Action Partner or Sponsor.
- Send an email to: phonebridgeoutreach@gmail.com for a list of Phone Numbers, Email addresses for Phone Buddies, Action Partners & Sponsors, and to volunteer to be a Phone Buddy, Action Partner or Sponsor.

What are the types of sponsors?
- Food Sponsor: Sponsors people who want to follow the requirements of the CEA-HOW method of refraining from compulsive eating.
- Inventory Sponsor: Sponsors people who want to read and learn about doing a Fourth Step Inventory, from various 4th Step materials, and to do the Inventory with a Sponsor, one-on-one.
- Step Sponsor: Sponsors people who want to read about discuss, and work though the practice of The Twelve Steps & Twelve Traditions with a Sponsor, one-on-one.
- Maintenance Sponsor: Sponsors people who are working a personal plan of recovery and want to maintain their recovery.
- Threefold Sponsor: Food, Inventory, Step, Maintenance: Physical, Emotional, Spiritual

Are there online email discussion groups?
- No

Does the organization have free meditations?
- No

Cups & Scales

cupsandscales-subscribe@yahoogroups.com

....

- "Cups & Scales" is an online discussion group
  cupsandscales-subscribe@yahoogroups.com
  started in 2010, to discuss weighing & measuring food and emotions.

  Over the years a practice has grown up where many people weigh and measure their food as part of a personal plan of recovery from compulsive overeating, food addiction, anorexia, bulimia, emotional eating and other eating disorders. There are many women and men recovering who DO NOT weigh and measure their food. The moderators take no position on weighing and measuring food. There are many strong feelings about it. This forum is neither endorsed by nor sponsored by any organization.

- 'Cups & Scales' takes its name from the book *Cups & Scales, Weighing & Measuring Food & Emotions* by Anonymous Twelve Step Recovery Members. This book is after the famous AA-book *Stools & Bottles* that discusses character defects of the alcoholic. Plus it contains information to contact people and groups who weigh and measure food, including people in *Compulsive Overeaters Anonymous-HOW; Cups & Scales Forum; Food Addicts Anonymous; Food Addicts: The Body Knows Online Discussion Group; Greysheeter's Anonymous; Overeaters Anonymous HOW and 90-Day meetings; and Recovery from Food Addiction*. Contacts are willing to be your phone buddy or to sponsor you. You get access to phone meeting numbers, websites, and email addresses to contact people who weigh and measure. The book is recommended literature.

  The compliment cookbook explains the "how to's" of weighing and measuring food. The contributors include no sugar-wheat-flour recipes and sample plans of eating with and without starches. *Cups & Scales Cookbook - Everything Weighed & Measured - Sample Plans of Eating & Recipes - No Sugar, Wheat, Flour - With & Without Starches & Grains* is recommended literature.
  Available at http://www.amazon.com

Food Addicts Anonymous, Inc.

http://www.foodaddictsanonymous.org/
561-967-3871

- "Food Addicts Anonymous Inc., founded in 1987, is a group of individuals helping one another, based on a belief that food addiction is a bio-chemical disease. By following a food plan devoid of all addictive substances, we can recover. These substances include sugar, flour, and wheat in all their forms. They also include fats and any other high-carbohydrate, refined, processed foods that cause us problems individually. You need to know that withdrawal is a necessary part of recovery. We can get better if we continue to follow our food plan, work the tools of the program, and ask for help.

"Food Addicts Anonymous is a fellowship of men and women who are willing to recover from the disease of food addiction. Sharing our experience, strength, and hope with others allows us to recover from this disease, one day at a time. Our primary purpose is to stay abstinent and to help other food addicts achieve abstinence. We invite you to join us on the road to recovery · and suggest you attend six meetings before you decide you don't need our help. Food Addicts Anonymous is self-supporting through our own contributions. We are not affiliated with any diet or weight loss programs, treatment facilities, or religious organizations. We neither endorse nor oppose any causes. Our primary purpose is to stay abstinent and to help other food addicts achieve abstinence. Food Addicts Anonymous was founded in December of 1987, by Judith C. in West Palm Beach, Florida
http://www.foodaddictsanonymous.org
website, May 2010."

There is an FAA plan of eating. It includes fruit, dairy, protein, vegetables, and starches and grains. People follow a food plan devoid of all addictive substances, including sugar, flour and wheat in all their forms. These substances also include fats and any other high-carbohydrate, refined, processed foods that cause problems individually. The FAA plan of eating is found on the website:
http://www.foodaddictsanonymous.org/faa-food-plan.

Are there phone meetings?
- Yes

How do I get a list of phone meetings?
- Click on http://www.foodaddictsanonymous.org/meetings-events
- To get started, dial 712-451-6000 PIN 7393#

  Sunday - 8 a.m., 9 a.m, 6 p.m., 10:30 p.m. EST

  Monday - 5:45 a.m., 10 a.m., 7 p.m., 9 p.m. 10:30 p.m. EST

  Tuesday - 5:45 a.m., 3 p.m., 8 p.m., 10 p.m. EST

  Wednesday - 5:45 a.m., 7 a.m., 11 a.m., 6:30 p.m., 10 p.m. EST

  Thursday - 5:45 a.m., 3 p.m., 9 p.m. EST

  Friday - 5:45 a.m., 11 a.m., 8 p.m., 10 p.m. EST

  Saturday - 8 a.m., 10 a.m., 8 p.m. EST

What are the types of phone meetings?

- Food for the Soul
- Newcomers
- Speaker
- Promises
- Tools
- Literature

Are there online meetings?
- Yes

How do I get a list of online meetings?
- Go to: http://www.foodaddictsanonymous.org/meetings-events

What are the types of online meetings?
- Phone Meeting and Chat Room On-Line Meetings
  Nationwide Meetings for FAA on the Web
- If you have Netscape or MS Internet Explorer, you can attend live FAA meetings in the FAA Chatroom. If you have AOL, you can also participate in the meetings.
- Meeting Days and Times
  FAA On-Line Regular Meetings
  Sundays 1pm EST and 10am PST
  FAA On-Line Beginners Meeting
  Saturday 11am EST and 8am PST

Are there face-to-face meetings?
- Yes

How do I get a list of face-to-face meetings?
- Click on: http://www.foodaddictsanonymous.org/meetings-events

What are the Types of face-to-face meetings?
- Face to face, two or more compulsive overeaters come together to share.

Are there sponsors, phone buddies & action partners?
- Yes

How do I get a sponsor, phone buddy or action partner?
How do I get a list of "We Care" phone numbers & email addresses, people willing to help?
- Ask for a Sponsor, Phone Buddy or Action Partner in FAA.org.
- Send a blank email to: FAA-Loop-subscribe@yahoogroups.com or

What are the types of sponsors, phone buddies & action partners?
- Threefold Sponsor: Food, Inventory, Step, Maintenance: Physical, Emotional, Spiritual.

Are there online email discussion groups?
- Yes

How do I get a list of online email discussion groups?
- Click on http://greenfaa.nfshost.com/forum/
- Online OA & 12 Step Recovery email discussion groups are hosted by • OA12StepforCOES • The Recovery Group • Food Addicts Anonymous • OA Primary Purpose • Recovery from Food Addiction (RFA) • The Body Knows. People go to the Discussion Group's website address from their Internet and join the discussion group by using their individual email to post and receive messages. Individuals will receive emails from the discussion group at the individual's email address. People may post, discuss, and talk to other members in response to topics and discussion in the discussion group through email responses to discussion group emails. The Recovery Group, OA12StepsforCOES, Food Addicts Anonymous, OA Primary Purpose, Recovery from Food Addiction (RFA) and The Body Knows email discussion groups are not affiliated with Overeaters Anonymous Inc.

Food Addiction: The Body Knows

http://www.kaysheppard.com/
kshepp825@aol.com
321-727-8040
thebodyknows-subscribe@yahoogroups.com

- "The Body Knows" thebodyknows-subscribe@yahoogroups.com is an online discussion group, with phone meetings, face-to-face meetings in Florida, and online meetings via online chat. It is a group of people who use the plan of eating suggested in the book Food Addiction: The Body Knows, 1989 by Kay Sheppard. Started in 2000, the group is open to everyone; there are no requirements to join the group. People discuss how to use a "Recovery Food Plan" suggested by Kay Sheppard with the principles of 12 Step Recovery; how to recognize the dangers in so-called "health" foods; how to overcome emotional barriers to recovery; how to find recovery buddies; how to recognize the warning signs of relapse; and how to incorporate the Twelve Steps into your life to stay motivated and achieve success.

   There is a suggested plan of eating. It includes fruit, dairy, protein, vegetables, and starches and grains. People follow a food plan devoid of all addictive substances, including sugar, flour and wheat in all their forms. These substances also include fats and any other high-carbohydrate, refined, processed foods that cause problems individually. is similar to the plan of eating recommended in Food Addicts Anonymous. It includes an additional serving of starch and grain at lunch. The plan of eating recommends no caffein, no sweeteners and weighed and measured servings. The plan of eating is found on the website: http://www.kaysheppard.com.

Are there online meetings?
- Yes

How do I get a list of online meetings?
- Go to: http://www.kaysheppard.com

What are the types of online meetings?
- Monday: 9:00 p.m. EST: Chat Room: http://www.kaysheppard.com
- Wednesday: 7:00 p.m. EST: Chat Room: http://www.kaysheppard.com
- Sunday: 8 p.m. EST: Chat Room: http://www.kaysheppard.com

Are there face-to-face meetings?
- Yes

How do I get a list of face-to-face meetings?
- Go to: http://www.kaysheppard.com

What are the Types of face-to-face meetings?
- Food Addiction: The Body Knows

Are there online email discussion groups?
- Yes

How do I get a list of online email discussion groups?
- To join "The Body Knows" send a blank email to: (thebodyknows-subscribe@yahoogroups.com The discussion group is a group of people who use the plan of eating suggested in the book Food Addiction: The Body Knows, 1989 by Kay Sheppard. Started in 2000, "Food Addiction: The Body Knows" is a website (http://www.kaysheppard.com and online discussion group operated by Kay Sheppard, nutritionist and food counselor.

Greysheeters Anonymous (GSA)

http://www.greysheet.org/cms/
GSA World Services or GSAWS, Inc.
Cherokee Station
PO Box 20098
New York, NY 10021-0061
uscontacts@greysheet.org
phonelist@greysheet.org

- Greysheeters Anonymous Inc., founded in 1998, is made up of individuals who strongly support the Greysheet Food Plan, weighing and measuring food, and communicating with a sponsor, as a method to recover from compulsive eating.

- "Greysheeters Anonymous is a fellowship of men and women who share their experience, strength, and hope with each other that they may solve their common problem and help others to recover from compulsive overeating. The group is open to everyone. The only requirement for membership is the desire to stop eating compulsively. There are no dues or fees for GSA membership; we are self-supporting through our own contributions. GSA is not allied with any sect, denomination, politics, organization, or institution; does not wish to engage in any controversy; neither endorses nor opposes any causes. Our primary purpose is to stay abstinent and help other compulsive overeaters to achieve abstinence. GreySheeters Anonymous has been founded and designed to discuss the fundamentals or basics of attaining and maintaining GreySheet abstinence. For that purpose we explore together the program of Alcoholics Anonymous in arresting compulsive eating. We strongly support GreySheet. We require that our meeting leaders be abstinent for at least three months on the GreySheet.

  We support a vigorous and positive attitude toward GreySheet abstinence which we define as three weighed and measured meals a day from the GreySheet, with nothing in between but black coffee, tea, or diet soda. A 'Greysheet Food Plan' may be obtained by first getting a Greysheet Sponsor. A qualified GreySheet sponsor is someone who has at least 90 days of back-to- back, uninterrupted GS abstinence. Greysheeters Anonymous Website, http://www.greysheet.org, May 2010.

A list of available sponsors is available from:
http://www.greysheet.org/cms/sponsors.html.

A sponsor explains how to weigh and measure without exception from the GreySheet Food Plan and provides a copy of the GreySheet Food Plan. GreySheet abstinence is defined by Greysheet Anonymous as: • Weighing and measuring three meals a day from the GreySheet as explained by a qualified GreySheet sponsor, • Committing those meals to a qualified GreySheet sponsor before eating them, • Doing this without exception, i.e., there is no situation where we do not weigh and measure, • Eating or drinking nothing in between those three meals except black coffee, black tea, no-calorie soft drinks, or water Greysheet Anonymous,

http://www.greysheet.org

- There is a required plan of eating. The Greysheet plan of eating comes with a Sponsor. The Greysheet food plan was originally offered for suggestion by Overeater's Anonymous Inc. in the 1960's, a very low carb, high protein food plan, no breads, flour products, only products that list sugar at least fifth on the label, and quantities suggested in weighed and measured amounts.

Are there online meetings?
- No

Are there phone meetings?
- Yes

How do I get a list of phone meetings?
- Go to: http://www.greysheet.org/cms/phone-meetings.html
- Send an email to: phonemeetings@greysheet.org for a list of phone meetings and PINS.

What are the types of phone meetings?
- 12 & 12
- AA Big Book
- AA Literature/Topic
- As Bill Sees It
- Beginners
- Literature
- Qualification/Speaker
- Relapse/Recovery
- Step Study

Are there face-to-face meetings?

- Yes

How do I get a list of face-to-face meetings?

- Go to: http://www.greysheet.org/cms/face-to-face-meetings.html

What are the types of face-to-face meetings?

- 12 & 12
- AA Big Book
- AA Literature/Topic
- As Bill Sees It
- Beginners
- Literature
- Living Sober
- Men's Meeting
- Qualification/Speaker
- Relapse/Recovery
- Step Study

Are there sponsors, phone buddies & action partners?

- Yes

How do I get a sponsor, phone buddy or action partner?
How do I get a list of "We Care" phone numbers & email addresses, people willing to help?

- Subscribe to this monthly list publication at:

  http://www.greysheet.org/cms/international-contacts.html, which lists hundreds of members worldwide, including available sponsors.
- Sponsors are available at: • Face-To-Face Meetings, • Phone Meetings, • Online - For initial contact only, to obtain a sponsor's phone number, • International Phone List.
- Join GreyNet - Post a request to this online group, to obtain a sponsor's phone number privately.
- To subscribe to the greynet, send a blank email to:

  greynet-subscribe@yahoogroups.com.
- Join Online Greysheeters Anonymous Forums:

  http://www.greysheet.org/forum/.

- Send an email to: phonelist@greysheet.org and uscontacts@greysheet.org
  for a list of Phone Numbers & Email addresses for Phone Buddies, Action Partners & Sponsors, and to volunteer to be a Phone Buddy, Action Partner or Sponsor. Provide your Name, Address, Phone Number(s), E-mail; Availablility to Sponsor. The list will only be provided to people who supply information. Privacy will be protected.

What are the types of sponsors, phone buddies & action partners?
- AA Big Book & 12 Steps Sponsor: Sponsors people who want to work through the AA Big Book and 12 Steps & 12 Traditions, by reading and discussing the materials, one-on-one.
- Food Sponsor: Sponsors people who want to discuss the Greysheet Food Plan and their food, weighing & measuring, and commit their food from the Greysheet before they eat it, to a Greysheet Sponsor, as a part of a personal plan of recovery.
- Inventory Sponsor: Sponsors people who want to read and learn about doing a Fourth Step Inventory, from various 4th Step materials, and to do the Inventory with a Sponsor, one-on-one.
- Maintenance Sponsor: Sponsors people who are working a personal plan of recovery and want to maintain their recovery.
- Step Sponsor: Sponsors people who want to read about, discuss, and work though the practice of The Twelve Steps & Twelve Traditions with a Sponsor, one-on-one.
- Weighing & Measuring Sponsor: Sponsors people who want to use cups & scales to weigh & measure food from a plan of eating as part of a personal plan of recovery. Many people share about using weighing and measuring as part of their personal plan of recovery, and volunteer to help people get started weighing and measuring from a plan of eating in many meetings.
- Threefold Sponsor: Food, Inventory, Step, Maintenance: Physical, Emotional,

Overeaters Anonymous Inc. (OA)

http://www.oa.org/
PO Box 44020
Rio Rancho, New Mexico 87174-4020 USA
http://www.oa.org/contact.php
505-891-2664

- "Overeaters Anonymous is a fellowship of individuals who, through shared experience, strength, and hope are recovering from compulsive eating and compulsive eating behaviors. There are no dues or fees for members; members are self-supporting through their own contributions, neither soliciting nor accepting outside donations. OA is not affiliated with any public or private organization, political movement, ideology, or religious doctrine; it takes no position on outside issues. OA's primary purpose is to abstain from compulsive eating and to carry the message of recovery to those who still suffer. The group is open to everyone. The only requirement for membership is a desire to stop eating compulsively.

- Who belongs to OA? In Overeaters Anonymous, you'll find members who are extremely overweight, even morbidly obese; moderately overweight; average weight; underweight; still maintaining periodic control; or totally unable to control their compulsive eating. OA members experience many different patterns of food behaviors. These 'symptoms' are as varied as our membership. Among them are: • obsession with body weight, size and shape • eating binges or grazing • preoccupation with reducing diets • starving • laxative or diuretic abuse • excessive exercise • inducing vomiting after eating • chewing and spitting out food • use of diet pills, shots and other medical interventions to control weight • inability to stop eating certain foods after taking the first bite • fantasies about food • vulnerability to quick-weight-loss schemes • constant preoccupation with food • using food as a reward or comfort. Our symptoms may vary, but OA participants share a common bond: we are powerless over food and our lives are unmanageable. This common problem has led those in OA to seek and find a common solution in the Twelve Steps, the Twelve traditions and eight tools of Overeaters Anonymous. The only requirement for membership is 'a desire to stop compulsively overeating.'

- Overeaters Anonymous neither endorses nor supports any specific plan of eating. The OA pamphlet 'Dignity of Choice' explains different plans of eating and recommends that an individual work with their nutritionist or healthcare practitioner in choosing a plan of eating as part of a personal plan of recovery.

- The organization's definition of abstinence is 'refraining from compulsive eating.' Face-to-face meetings, phone meetings, and online meetings are open to everyone"(Overeaters Anonymous Inc, 2010, http://www.oa.org).

Are there phone meetings?
- Yes

How do I get a list of phone meetings?
- Click on http://www.oa.org/pdfs/phone_mtgs.pdf
  for a Printed List of OA Phone Meetings"
- Go to http://www.oa.org. Click on Meetings.
  Click on Telephone. Set your Time Zone; Print Phone Meeting List
- Over 150 OA Phone Meetings a Week

What are the types of phone meetings?
- AA 12 Step Steps & Traditions - Focuses on reading from the AA 12 Steps & Traditions and discussing each step and tradition in relation to compulsive eating.
- Anorexia-Bulemia - Focuses on starving, restricting, purging and diet remedies as compulsive behaviors to deal with compulsive eating.
- Beginner/Newcomer - Focuses on an introduction to the Steps & Traditions and Tools of OA for the Newcomer; how to get a Sponsor, Phone Buddy or Action Partner, and OA resources.
- Big Book - Focuses on reading and discussing The AA Big Book.

- 90 Day* - Meetings giving help to people who want a structured approach, including weighing and measuring, calling a Sponsor daily, making three outreach calls daily, and 90 days abstinence to share on phone meetings.

- OA H.O.W* - "H.O.W. is a movement within Overeaters Anonymous whose basic principle is that abstinence is the only means to freedom from compulsive overeating and the beginning of a spiritual life. We believe that the discipline of weighing and measuring, of telephoning your sponsor at a particular time, of attending meetings and making phone calls; all lead to a life based on the Universal Discipline, which is accord rather than discord even with many things going on around us. • We eat weighed and measured meals with nothing in between except sugar free beverages and sugar free gum. • Food is written down, called in to our sponsor and committed, so that we can get on with our recovery and out of the food. • We do not write our own food plan. We use a food plan given to us by a doctor, nutritionist or dietician. We discuss it with our sponsor. We do not pick one that allows any of our binge foods. If some food on our plan becomes a problem, we avoid it. • We do not skip meals, switch meals or combine eals. We do not deviate or manipulate our food plan in any way. If we need to change our committed food during the day, we call a sponsor. • We weigh and measure all our portions so that there is no guess work. We do not measure by eye. We use a measuring cup, spoon, and a scale. • We weigh ourselves once a month until we reach goal weight and once a week on maintenance. • Unless advised otherwise by your doctor, we take a multi-vitamin and drink 64 oz. of water a day. • We do not drink alcohol. • We do not use foods containing sugar, except if sugar is listed 5th or beyond on the ingredients label. • A H.O.W. sponsor is a compulsive overeater who has completed at least 70 days of back-to-back abstinence and who has taken the first three steps of the

program. Sponsors have also completed at least 70 days of assignments. • In HOW we are asked to make at least 4 telephone calls a day; one to our sponsor and 3 more to other OA members. These calls give us an opportunity to "talk program" on a daily basis. • As H.O.W. members we attend at least one H.O.W. meeting a week." (OA H.O.W. Statement, March 2010).

- One Hundred Pounders- 100 Pounders - Focuses on recovery for people who have lost or want to lose 100 pounds or more
- Relapse/Recovery 12th Step Within - Literarure/discussion from 12th Step Within
- Seeking the Spiritual Path - Literature/discussion on Seeking the Spiritual Path
- Speaker/Qualification - A Speaker will share his/her Experience, Strength, Hope on recovery.
- Topic/Discussion - Moderator will set a topic for discussion.
- Voices of Recovery - Literature/discussion Voices of Recovery
- Weighing & Measuring* – OA 90 Day and OA H.O.W. meetings suggest weighing and measuring food as part of a structured approach to being released from compulsive eating.
- Young People/Everyone - Topic/Discussion with Young People/Everyone

....

Are there all day phone marathons?
- Holiday Marathons: from 6:45 a.m. EST to Midnight EST, Continuously Every Hour.
- OA Special Day Phone Marathons

....

How do I get a list of marathon phone meetings dates & times?
- Holiday Marathons:
  from 6:45 a.m. EST to Midnight EST, Continuously Every Hour.
- Send a blank email to oaphonemarathons-subscribe@yahoogroups.com for a list of OA • Special Day Phone Marathons

....

Are there online meetings?
- Yes

....

How do I get a list of online meetings?
- Click on: http://www.oa.org/pdfs/onlinemeetingslist.pdf for a pdf Printed List of Online Meetings
- Go to: http://www.oa.org/meetings/find-a-meeting-online.php for a complete list of OA Online Meetings
- Go to http://www.therecoverygroup.org/newcomers.html and click the doorway, to see OA meetings registered with OA World Services

- Go to: http://oa12step4coes.org for a list of online meeting times and days, for online OA meetings sponsored by this OA Intergroup.
- Online OA meetings are held by • Overeaters Anonymous Inc. • The Recovery Group • OA12StepforCOES at website addresses. The Online meetings take place through Online Chat or Online SKYPE telephone. The meetings follow a meeting format. The Recovery Group online meetings are not affiliated with Overeaters Anonymous Inc.

What are the types of online meetings?
- AA Big Book
- Beginner/Newcomer
- Hebrew
- Italian
- OA H.O.W.
- Spanish
- 12 Steps & 12 Traditions

Are there face-to-face meetings?
- Yes

How do I get a list of face-to-face meetings?
- Go to http://www.oa.org
  Click on Meetings in Upper Righthand corner or Lefthand Navigation Bar;

What are the types of face-to-face meetings?
- AA 12 Step Steps & Traditions - Focuses on reading from the AA 12 Steps & Traditions and discussing each step and tradition in relation to compulsive eating.
- Anorexia-Bulimia - Focuses on starving, restricting, purging and diet remedies as compulsive behaviors to deal with compulsive eating.
- Beginner/Newcomer - Focuses on an introduction to the Steps & Traditions and Tools of OA for the Newcomer; how to get a Sponsor, Phone Buddy or Action Partner, and OA resources.
- Big Book - Focuses on reading and discussing The AA Big Book with reference to compulsive eating.

- 90 Day* - Meetings giving help to people who want a structured approach, including weighing and measuring, calling a Sponsor daily, making three outreach calls daily, and 90 days abstinence to share on phone meetings.
- OA 12 Steps & Traditions- Focuses on the OA 12 Steps & Traditions.
- OA H.O.W* - "H.O.W. is a movement within Overeaters Anonymous whose basic principle is that abstinence is the only means to freedom from compulsive overeating and the beginning of a spiritual life. We believe that the discipline of weighing and measuring, of telephoning your sponsor at a particular time, of attending meetings and making phone calls; all lead to a life based on the Universal Discipline, which is accord rather than discord even with many things going on around us. • We eat weighed and measured meals with nothing in between except sugar free beverages and sugar free gum. • Food is written down, called in to our sponsor and committed, so that we can get on with our recovery and out of the food. • We do not write our own food plan. We use a food plan given to us by a doctor, nutritionist or dietician. We discuss it with our sponsor. We do not pick one that allows any of our binge foods. If some food on our plan becomes a problem, we avoid it. • We do not skip meals, switch meals or combine meals.
manipulate our food plan in any way. If we need to change our committed food during the day, we call a sponsor. • We weigh and measure all our portions so that there is no guess work. We do not measure by eye. We use a measuring cup, spoon, and a scale. • We weigh ourselves once a month until we reach goal weight and once a week on maintenance. • Unless advised otherwise by your doctor, we take a multi-vitamin and drink 64 oz. of water a day. • We do not drink alcohol. • We do not use foods containing sugar, except if sugar is listed 5th or beyond on the ingredients label. • A H.O.W. sponsor is a compulsive overeater who has completed at least 70 days of back-to-back abstinence and who has taken the first three steps of the program. Sponsors have also completed at least 70 days of assignments. • In HOW we are asked to make at least 4 telephone calls a day; one to our sponsor and 3 more to other OA members. These calls give us an opportunity to "talk program" on a daily basis. • As H.O.W. members we attend at least one H.O.W. meeting a week." (OA H.O.W. Statement, March 2010).
- One Hundred Pounders- 100 Pounders - Focuses on recovery for people who have lost or want to lose 100 pounds or more
- Relapse/Recovery 12th Step Within - Literarure/discussion from 12th Step Within
- Seeking the Spiritual Path - Literature/discussion on Seeking the Spiritual Path
- Speaker/Qualification - A Speaker will share his/her Experience, Strength, Hope on recovery.
- Traditions Study - Literature/discussion on 12 Traditions
- Weighing & Measuring* – OA 90 Day and OA H.O.W. meetings suggest weighing and measuring food as part of a structured approach to being released from compulsive eating.

Are there sponsors, phone buddies & action partners?
- Yes

How do I get a sponsor, phone buddy or action partner?
How do I get a list of "We Care" phone numbers & email addresses, people willing to help?
- Sponsors, Phone Buddies & Action Partners are available at: • Face-To-Face Meetings, • Phone Meetings, • Online Meetings • From "We Care" Phone Number & Email lists • By eMail or Mail.
- The "We Care" list is a list of people who have shared their phone numbers or emails to receive and give OA outreach contact. • Ask if the meeting has a "We Care" list. • Look at the "We Care" list and write down names and numbers. • Email for the "We Care" list at the email addresses given. Ask at a Phone Meeting, Face-to-Face Meeting, Online Meeting or Email Discussion Group for a Sponsor, Phone Buddy or Action Partner.
- Send a blank email to: oa645business-subscribe@yahoogroups.com to join. Once you have joined, go to the group at: http://www.yahoogroups.com/. Click on Files. You will see a PDF list of Phone Numbers & Email addresses, for Phone Buddies, Action Partners & Sponsors, and to volunteer to be a Phone Buddy, Action Partner or Sponsor from the 6:45 a.m. Sunrise Meeting.
- Send an email to: recoveryinaction@yahoo.com for a list of Phone Numbers & Email addresses, for Phone Buddies, Action Partners & Sponsors, and to volunteer to be a Phone Buddy, Action Partner or Sponsor from the OA H.O.W meeting.
- Send an email to: fortodaylunchtimemeeting@gmail.com for a list of Phone Numbers & Email addresses for Phone Buddies, Action Partners & Sponsors, and to volunteer to be a Phone Buddy, Action Partner or Sponsor from 12:00 Lunchtime meeting EST.
- Send an email to: pianosheila@yahoo.com or call Sheila P. at (303) 980-1664 for a list of Phone Numbers & Email addresses for Phone Buddies, Action Partners & Sponsors, and to volunteer to be a Phone Buddy, Action Partner or Sponsor from the 8:30 a.m. OA 90-Day Program
- Send an email to 100pounders@gmail for a list of Phone Numbers & Email addresses for Phone Buddies, Action Partners & Sponsors and to volunteer for outreach from the 100 Pounders meeting.
- Send an email to: Sponsors@TheRecoveryGroup.org for a list Phone Numbers & Email addresses for Phone Buddies, Action Partners & Sponsors, and to volunteer to be a Phone Buddy, Action Partner or Sponsor from The Recovery Group - OA . Read about The Recovery Group Sponsor Program at: http://www.therecoverygroup.org/sponsors.html.

- Are you a Loner? Phone Buddies, Action Partners & Sponsors are available for Loners. Are you living in a remote area, away from nearby 12 Step meetings?
- Click http://www.oaregion10.org/PDFs/loners.pdf for some loner OA member outreach stories - Loner Stories.
- Click http://www.oa.org and complete the online form: http://www.oa.org/pdfs/sbm_form.pdf for the OA World Service Office by Mail program, or email the World Service Office at info@oa.org. for support by mail or email. Or write directly to OA at: OA, PO Box 44020, Rio Rancho, NM 87174-4020 USA. Or identify your Region (see Regions below for U.S. States and Countries in regions 1-10).

What are the types of sponsors, phone buddies & action partners?
- AA Big Book & 12 Steps Sponsor: Sponsors people who want to work through the AA Big Book and 12 Steps & 12 Traditions, by reading and discussing the materials, one-on-one.
- eMail Sponsor - Sponsors people who want to maintain an e-mail connection, writing to the sponsor on a regular basis, either their food food or ways they are working a program.
- Food Sponsor: sponsors people who want to discuss their food as a part of a personal plan of recovery.
- Inventory Sponsor: Sponsors people who want to read and learn about doing a Fourth Step Inventory, from various 4th Step materials, and to do the Inventory with a Sponsor, one-on-one.
- Maintenance Sponsor: Sponsors people who are working a personal plan of recovery and want to maintain their recovery.
- 90-Day Meeting Sponsor - Sponsors people who are working the 90 Day Program. The 90-Day program recommends weighing & measuring food from a plan of eating as part of a personal plan of recovery & making outreach phone calls. Attend a 90-Day Phone Meeting to listen to the suggestions advised in the 90-Day program and to get a 90-Day Meeting Sponsor.
- OA H.O.W. Sponsor - "A H.O.W. sponsor is a compulsive overeater who has completed at least 70 days of back-to-back abstinence and who has taken the first three steps of the program. Sponsors have also completed at least 70 days of assignments. • In HOW we are asked to make at least 4 telephone calls a day; one to our sponsor and 3 more to other OA members. These calls give us an opportunity to "talk program" on a daily basis. • As H.O.W. members we attend at least one H.O.W. meeting a week.

Recovery from Food Addiction (RFA)

recoveryfromfoodaddiction-subscribe@yahoogroups.com
P.O. Box 35543
713-673-2848

There are no requirements to join the online group. People discuss how to use a "Recovery Food Plan" suggested by Kay Sheppard (www.kaysheppard.com) with the principles of 12 Step Recovery.

There is a suggested plan of eating. It includes fruit, dairy, protein, vegetables, and starches and grains. People follow a food plan devoid of all addictive substances, including sugar, flour and wheat in all their forms. These substances include fats and any other high carbohydrate, refined, processed foods that cause problems individually. The Recovery from Food Addiction food plan is similar to the plan of eating recommended in Food Addicts Anonymous; the RFA plan includes an additional serving of starch and grain at lunch.

Are there online meetings?
- No

Are there phone meetings?
- Yes

How do I get a list of phone meetings?
- To get started dial 218-339-4300 PIN 1086405#
  Friday Night @ 9:00 pm EST

What are the types of phone meetings?
- Recovery from Food Addiction

Are there all day phone marathons?
- No

Are there sponsors, phone buddies & action partners?

- Yes

How do I get a sponsor, phone buddy or action partner?
How do I get a list of "We Care" phone numbers & email addresses, people willing to p?

- Subscribe to: recoveryfromfoodaddiction-subscribe@yahoogroups.com for Phone Buddies, Action Partners & Sponsors, and to volunteer to be a Phone Buddy, Action Partner or Sponsor.

- Sponsors are available at meetings and from a "We Care" Phone Number and Email list, for a Sponsor, Phone Buddy, Action Partner or other form of help. Ask at a meeting for a Sponsor, Phone Buddy or Action Partner. Ask if a meeting has a "We Care" list. Look at the "We Care" list to see the individuals giving their Phone Number or Email contact information for outreach. Sponsors are available at: • Face-To-Face Meetings, • Phone Meetings, • From "We Care" Phone Number & Email lists

What are the types of sponsors, phone buddies & action partners?

- AA Big Book & 12 Steps Sponsor: Sponsors people who want to work through the AA Big Book and 12 Steps & 12 Traditions, by reading and discussing the materials.

Are there online email discussion groups?

- Yes

How do I get a list of online email discussion groups?

- Subscribe to: recoveryfromfoodaddiction-subscribe@yahoogroups.com to join.
- Online OA & 12 Step Recovery email discussion groups are hosted by • OA12StepforCOES • The Recovery Group • OA Primary Purpose • Recovery from Food Addiction (RFA) • The Body Knows. People go to the Discussion Group's website address from their Internet and join the discussion group by using their individual email to post and receive messages. Individuals will receive emails from the discussion group at the individual's email address. People may post, discuss, and talk to other members in response to topics and discussion in the dicscussion group through email responses to discussion group emails. The Recovery Group, OA12StepsforCOES, OA Primary Purpose, Recovery from Food Addiction (RFA) and The Body Knows email discussion groups are not affiliated with Overeaters Anonymous Inc

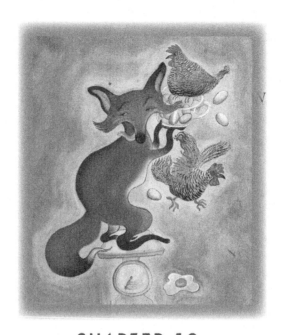

CHAPTER 10
Sweeteners
Each One Makes a Decision

This cookbook does not use sugar or other forms of sugar in recipes. A recipe may say sweetener (optional). Each person must decide for themselves on the use of sweeteners -- whether they are going to use sweeteners, on what occasions, how much sweetness, whether the use will be sweeteners that are other forms of sugar or artificial sweeteners made from chemicals only, in what amounts, or if at all.

Sweeteners or sugar substitutes are used
1. by the food industry because their cost is less than the cost of sugar,
2. by the food industry because the level of sweetness is greater than the sweetness provided by sugar,
3. by individuals with diabetes mellitus who want to limit their sugar intake,
4. by people with hypoglycemia who create an excess of insulin after quickly absorbing glucose into the bloodstream,
5. by individuals who want to limit their food energy caloric intake by replacing high caloric high energy value sugar foods with low-energy or no-energy no caloric sweeteners. Here is a brief history of sugar and a partial list of various names for sweeteners.

A Brief History of Sugar ~ Sugar Substitutes ~ Sweeteners

Before 1650, there was no 'table sugar' in America, England or the rest of the world. Imagine. Table sugar came as ships sailed from Europe to the Caribbean Islands with the Trade Winds across the Atlantic, and picked up refined cane sugar, slaves, and rum, (Sweetness & Power, Sidney Mintz).

The ships sailed north to America on the Trade Winds and carried the cargo, bringing the sugar, slaves and rum to America. Then the ships sailed on the Trade Winds back across the Atlantic, bringing the cane sugar to the tables in England. There was a time before people put table sugar in their tea, before sugar bowls, and before the many confections made with refined table sugar. (Sweetness& Power, Sidney Mintz)

The market price of the commodity sugar has not declined in three centuries. The taste for "sweetness" has grown around the world. The taste buds for sweetness are built in to our evolutionary history. They insured that we would gravitate in our distant past to foods that had sucrose for energy and survival.

The taste for sugar created new industries around the world. Refined sugar was at first the luxury of the aristocracy who showed wealth in their display of confections such as fancy cakes. Gradually increased manufacture made sugar available to the masses as a cheap source of calories.

The taste for "sweetness" created a new market for "sweeter" products. "Sweetness" was sold. New agricultural and chemical manufacturing methods created a means for producing "sweetness" under other names for sugar. These chemical forms of sweetness could be manufactured less expensively than refined sugar. They now compete with sugar cane on the world market as an ingredient additive because they are less expensive as an additive than cane sugar. (RuddCenter/Yale for Obesity & Food Addictions, http://www.ruddcenteryale.org).

The food and beverage industry is increasingly replacing sugar with HFCS, high fructose corn syrup and with artificial sweeteners in a range of products traditionally containing sugar. a fraction of the cost of natural sweeteners. (Wikipedia,http://www.wikipedia.com). Aspartame is currently the most popular sweetener in the U.S. food industry, as the price has dropped significantly since the Monsanto Company patent expired in 1992. However, sucralose may soon replace it, as alternative processes to Tate & Lyle's patent seem to be emerging. According to Morgan Stanley, this can mean that the price of sucralose will drop by 30%. (Fletcher, Anthony, 2006).

MAJOR TYPES & CHEMISTRY OF SWEETENERS

A sweetener is a food additive that duplicates the effect of sugar in taste, usually with less food energy. Some sweeteners are known either as sugar substitutes (natural, meaning made from sugar or an ingredient grown in nature) and some are synthetic (made from chemicals alone). (Wikipedia, http://www.wikipedia.com).

SWEETENERS: OTHER FORMS OF SUGAR (MADE FROM SUGAR OR AN INGREDIENT GROWN IN NATURE)

Adenylic Acid or Adenosine
Monophosphate (AMP)
Brazzein
Curculin
Erythritol
Glycyrrhizin
Glycerol
Hydrogenated starch
Inulin
Isomalt
Lactitol
Luo Han Guo
Mabinlin
Maltitol
Maltooligosaccharide
Mannitol
Miraculin
Monatin
Monellin
Pentadin
Sorbitol
Stevia
Tagatose
Thaumatin
Xylitol
Xylitol
(Wikipedia, http://www.wikipedia.com).

OTHER NAMES FOR SUGAR:

Barbados Sugar
Barley Malt
Beet Juice
Beet Sugar Cane Sugar
Black Strap Molasses Cane Syrup Brown
Rice Syrup (In Most Soy Caramel Milks)
Carob Powder
Brown Sugar Confectioner's Sugar
Cooked Honey Light Brown Sugar
Corn Starch Light Sugar
Corn Sugar Light Syrup

Corn Sweetener Lite Syrup
Corn Syrup Lo-Sugar
Corn Syrup
Crystalline Carbohydrate Low Sugar
Crystalline Fructose Malt
Dark Brown Sugar Malt Syrup
Date Sugar Malted
Date Syrup Malted Barley
Demerara (British) Malted Syrup
Dextrin Maltitol
Dextrose Malto-(Anything Else)
Disaccharides Maltodextrin
Evaporated/Crystallized Cane Juice
Maltose (Malt Sugar)
Fig Syrup Manitol
Filtered Honey Mannitol
Fructose Maple Sugar
Fruit Juice Concentrate (All Types)
Maple Syrup
Fruit Nectars Molasses
Fruit Sugar Mono-Saccharides
Fruit Sweetener Muscavado (Barbados
Sugar)
Galactose Natural Sweeteners
Glucose Natural Syrup
Golden Brown Sugar Polysaccharides
Granulated Sugar Poly-Saccharides
Grape Sugar Powdered Sugar
Grape Sweetener Raisin Syrup
Heavy Syrup Raw Honey
HFCS Raw Sugar
High Fructose Corn Syrup
Raw Sugar or Turbinado Sugar
Honey Ribbon Cane Syrup
Hydrogenated Glucose Syrup Ribose
Invert Sugar Rice Malts
 Jaggery Rice Syrup
Juice Concentrate Rum

Lactose (Milk Sugar) Sorghum
Levulose (Fruit Sugar) Sorghum
Molasses
Light Brown Sugar Light Sugar
Light Syrup
Lite Syrup Lo-Sugar Low Sugar
Malt
Malt Syrup Malted
Malted Barley
Malted Syrup
Maltitol Malto-(Anything Else)
Maltodextrin
Maltose (Malt Sugar)
Manitol
Mannitol
Maple Sugar
Maple Syrup
Molasses
Mono-Saccharides
Muscavado (Barbados Sugar)
Natural Syrup
Natural Sweeteners
Polydextrose
Polysaccharides
Poly-Saccharides
Powdered Sugar
Raisin Syrup
Raw Honey
Raisin Syrup
Raw Sugar
Raw Sugar or Turbinado Sugar
Ribbon Cane Syrup
Ribose
Rice Malts
Rice Syrup
Rum Sorghum Syrup
Starch Syrup
Stevia

Succanat
Sucrose (Table Sugar)
Sugar
Sugar Alcohols (Ex. Mannitol, Sorbitol,
Xylitol)
Sugar Cane Syrup
Syrups (Ex. Maple, Sorghum)
Table Sugar
Turbinado
Uncooked Honey
White Sugar
Xylitol

SWEETENERS: ARTIFICIAL SWEETENERS
(SYNTHETIC, MADE FROM CHEMICALS ONLY)

An important class of sugar substitutes are known as high-intensity sweeteners. These are compounds with sweetness that is many times that of sucrose, common table sugar. As a result, much less sweetener is required, and energy contribution often negligible. The sensation of sweetness caused by these compounds (the "sweetness profile") is sometimes notably different from sucrose, so they are often used in complex mixtures that achieve the most natural sweet sensation. If the sucrose (or other sugar) replaced has contributed to the texture of the product, then a bulking agent is often also needed. This may be seen in soft drinks labeled as "diet" or "light," which contain artificial sweeteners and often have notably different mouthfeel, or in table sugar replacements that mix maltodextrins with an intense sweetener to achieve satisfactory texture sensation (Wikipedia, http://www.wikipedia.com).

In the United States, six intensely-sweet sugar substitutes have been approved for use. They are **saccharin (e.g., Sweet'N Low), aspartame, sucralose, neotame, acesulfame potassium, and stevia.** There is some ongoing controversy over whether artificial sweetener usage poses health risks. (Wikipedia, http://www.wikipedia.com).

The US Food and Drug Administration regulates artificial sweeteners as food additives (Food & Drug Administration, 2006) Food Additives must be approved by the FDA, which publishes a Generally Recognized as Safe (GRAS) list of additives (Food & Drug Administration, "FDA Website Guidance Documents"). To date, the FDA has not been presented with scientific information that would support a change in conclusions about the safety of the six approved artificial sweeteners. The safe conclusions are based on a detailed review of a large body of information, including hundreds of toxicological and clinical studies (Food & Drug Administration, 2006).

There is also an herbal supplement, stevia, used as a sweetener. Controversy surrounds lack of research on stevia's safety and there is a battle over its approval as a sugar substitute (Columbia Daily Tribune, March 23, 2008). The majority of sugar substitutes approved for food use are artificially-synthesized compounds. However, some bulk natural sugar substitutes are known, including sorbitol and xylitol, which are found in berries, fruit, vegetables, and mushrooms. It is not commercially viable to extract these products from fruits and vegetables, so they

For example, xylose is converted to xylitol, lactose to lactitol, and glucose to sorbitol. Still other natural substitutes are known, but are yet to gain official approval for food use. Some non-sugar sweeteners are polyols, also known as "sugar alcohols." These are, in general, less sweet than sucrose, but have similar bulk properties and can be used in a wide range of food products. Sometimes the sweetness profile is 'fine-tuned' by mixing high-intensity sweeteners. As with all food products, the development of a formulation to replace sucrose is a complex proprietary process.

The three primary compounds used as sugar substitutes in the United States are SACCHARIN (E.G., SWEET'N LOW); ASPARTAME (E.G., EQUAL, NUTRASWEET); and SUCRALOSE (E.G., SPLENDA, ALTERN). In many other countries xylitol, cyclamate and the herbal sweetener stevia are used extensively. A sugar substitute is a food additive that duplicates the effect of sugar in taste, but usually has less food energy. Some sugar substitutes

SACCHARIN (E.G., SWEET'N LOW) Aside from sugar of lead, saccharin (e.g., Sweet'N Low) was the first artificial sweetener and was originally synthesized in 1879 by Remsen and Fahlberg. Its sweet taste was discovered by accident. It had been created in an experiment with toluene derivatives. A process for the creation of saccharin from phthalic anhydride was developed in 1950, and, currently, saccharin is created by this process as well as the original process by which it was discovered. It is 300 to 500 times as sweet as sugar (sucrose) and is often used to improve the taste of toothpastes, dietary foods, and dietary beverages. The bitter aftertaste of saccharin is often minimized by blending it with other sweeteners. Fear about saccharin increased when a 1960 study showed that high levels of saccharin may cause bladder cancer in laboratory rats. Subsequently, it was discovered that saccharin causes cancer in male rats by a mechanism not found in humans. In 2001, the United States repealed the warning label requirement, while the threat of an FDA ban had already been lifted in 1991. Most other countries also permit saccharin but restrict the levels of use, while other countries have outright banned it (Wikipedia, http://www.wikipedia.com).

ASPARTAME (E.G., EQUAL, NUTRASWEET) Aspartame was discovered in 1965 by James M. Schlatter at the G.D. Searle company (later purchased by Monsanto). He was working on an anti-ulcer drug and spilled some aspartame on his hand by accident. When he licked his finger, he noticed that it had a sweet taste. It is an odorless, white crystalline powder that is derived from the two amino acids aspartic acid and phenylalanine. It is about 200 times as sweet as sugar and can be used as a tabletop a sweetener or in frozen desserts, gelatins, beverages, and chewing gum. When eaten, aspartame is metabolized into its original amino acids and has a relatively low food energy. Since the FDA approved aspartame for consumption, some researchers have suggested that a rise in brain tumor rates in the United States may be at least partially related to the increasing availability and consumption of aspartame (Olney, J.W., Farber, N.B., Spitznagel E, Robins LN, November 1996).

Sucralose (e.g. Splenda) Sucralose (e.g., Splenda) is a chlorinated sugar that is about 600 times as sweet as sugar. It is ed in beverages, frozen desserts, chewing gum, baked goods, and other foods. Unlike other artificial sweeteners, it is stable when heated and can therefore be used in baked and fried goods. Sucralose is minimally absorbed by the body and most of it passes out of the body unchanged (Daniel J.W., Renwick A.G., Roberts A., Sims J., 2000). The FDA approved sucralose in 1998 (Food and Drug Administration, 1998). Most of the controversy surrounding Splenda, a sucralose sweetener, is focused not on safety, but on its marketing. It has been marketed with the slogan, "Splenda is made from sugar, so it tastes like sugar." Sucralose is a chlorinated sugar prepared from either sucrose or raffinose. With either base sugar, processing replaces three oxygen-hydrogen groups in the sugar molecule with three chlorine atoms (Wanjek, Christopher, May 2007).

Weight Gain or Weight Loss Properties of Sugar Substitutes & Artificial Sweeteners

A 2005 study by the University of Texas Health Science Center at San Antonio showed that increased weight gain and obesity was associated with increased use of diet soda in a population based study. The study did not establish whether increased weight leads to increased consumption of diet drinks or whether consumption of diet drinks could have an effect on weight gain (DeNoon, Daniel J. Reviewed by Charlotte Grayson Mathis MD., 2005). Animal studies have indicated that artificial sweeteners can cause body weight gain. A sweet taste induces an insulin response, which causes blood sugar to be stored in tissues (including fat), but because blood sugar does not increase with artificial sugars, there is hypoglycemia and increased food intake the next time there is a meal. After a while, rats given sweeteners have steadily increased calorie intake, increased body weight, and increased adiposity (fatness). Animals may use sweet taste to predict the caloric contents of food. Eating sweet non-caloric substances may degrade this predictive relationship. Plus, the natural responses to eating sugary foods (eating less at the next meal and using some of the extra calories to warm the body after the sugary meal) are gradually lost (Swithers S.E., Davidson T.L., 2008).

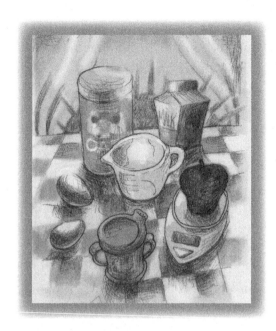

CHAPTER 11
Resources & Links

SCALES & CUPS

DIGITAL SCALES – MEASURING CUPS – MEASURING SPOONS

Amazon.com – http://www.amazon.com
Ebay.com – http://www.ebay.com
Pfaltzgraff.com, http://www.pfaltzgraff.com
Old Will Knott's Scales - http://www.oldwillknott.com/
MyScale.com - ScaleWorks, Gram Precision, Ohaus brands;
Call 866-222-2291. http://www.myscale.com/
American Weigh - American Weigh, Escali, Ohaus, Salter, Tanita -
http://www.americanweigh.com/

OIL MIST SPRAY PUMPS &
PRESS & MEASURE OIL DISPENSERS

NON-AEROSOL OIL MIST SPRAY PUMPS

A non-aerosol mister uses a pump to build up pressure and then sprays a fine mist of whatever oil is in it. Fill a container with your favorite oil, pump cap to pressurize & spray a thin film directly on the pan for non-stick, low-fat cooking. You can fill the container with herbs for color and flavor. You can create your own flavored oils by infusing oil with dried herbs, dried spices or even ingredients like dried chili peppers, sun dried tomatoes and dried garlic without clogging the sprayer. You can wash and sterilize a glass or aluminum mist container. This is perfect for misting salads and cooking pans.

We suggest you test for yourself the quantity your mister sprays – per mists. Take your mister, in a bowl, mist starting with 5 mists. Pour the mists into a teaspoon. See what the number of mists is you're your mister to equal 1 tsp. Many stores carry many different brands of oil mist sprayers.

Amazon.com – http://www.amazon.com
Ebay.com – http://www.ebay.com
Pfaltzgraff.com - http://www.pfaltzgraff.com
CrateandBarrel.com – http://www.crateandbarrel.com
Tabletop Mister
Cuisipro Stainless Steel Spray Non-Aerosol Mister
Misto Oil Bottle Sprayer

AEROSOL CAN COOKING SPRAY – ZERO-CALORIE-FAT FREE LABELING CLAIMS VS. FACTS

Aerosol cooking sprays are not fat free or zero-calorie. Aerosol cooking sprays DO NOT have to list fat ingredients on the label as long as there is 0.5 grams of fat – that is the amount estimated in a 1/3 second spray. When was the last time you sprayed something for a 1/3 second? A one second spray is about 7 calories of fat. Aerosol cooking sprays also contain emulsifiers, lecithin, and CFA's to create the aerosol propellant.

PRESS & MEASURE OIL DISPENSERS

Press and Measure oil dispenser pumps allow you to measure and pour the exact amount of oil to add to your recipe . You can pump from 1 tsp. to 2 tbs., see it in the top glass of the container, and pour the exact amount into the recipe. No overflow. This is perfect for "seeing" what 1 tsp. – 2 tbs. looks like "up close" in the top glass - then pouring the measured amount in the food. It creates a "look and see" "pause."

Many stores carry many different brands of press and measure oil dispenser pumps.

Ebay.com – http://www.ebay.com
Elementalkitchen.com – http://www.elementalkitchen.com
Amazon.com – http://www.amazon.com
Pfaltzgraff.com - http://www.pfaltzgraff.com
CrateandBarrel.com – http://www.crateandbarrel.com

Elemental Kitchen's Pump and Measure Oil / Vinegar Dispenser
Press & Measure Oil Dispenser at www.ebay.com

SOY PRODUCTS

I.M. Healthy Soy Nut Butter -http://www.soynutbutter.com/
Healthy Eating - http://www.healthy-eating.com/
Something Better Natural Foods - http://www.somethingbetternaturalfoods.com/
NOW Foods -http://www.nowfoods.com/

SOY PRODUCT DESCRIPTIONS:
NO SUGAR-NO FLOUR-NO FILLERS

Edamame, Fresh Green Soybeans - similar to green peas; available in pods or already shelled; usually frozen, but sometimes available fresh in Asian stores.
Seapoint Farms -http://www.seapointfarms.com/
Sunrich - http://www.sunrich.com
Melissa's World Variety Produce -http://www.melissas.com

Miso - aged and fermented soybean paste - sort of like solid soy sauce - great for flavoring tofu. Like tempeh, it is often mixed with grains, so becareful to get "hacho" miso - just the soybeans.

Soy Beans - black and white; hot or cold; dried that need soaking and cooking, or already cooked in cans.
Westbrae - http://www.westbrae.com
makes canned, organic soybeans. Just open and rinse the gel off with hot water.
Eden Foods -http://www.edenfoods.com/
makes canned, black organic soybeans.

Soy Bran - so far only found in the UK and delivered to the US by kind English folk. Only ingredient is soy. May be used in combination with oat meal or oat bran.

Soy Cheese - varieties that contain casein include:
Yves Veggie - http://www.yvesveggie.com/
Since casein is a protein from the lining of calves stomachs, most soy cheese is not vegan.

Soy Cream Cheese, Soy Cottage Cheese, Soy Sour Cream, and Soy Yogurt -
all seem to have casein. Since casein is a protein from the lining of calves stomachs, most soy cheese is not vegan.

Soy Milk - soaked, cooked soybeans that are ground, pressed, and filtered into a milk. Unopened, aseptically packaged soymilk can be stored at room temperature for several months. Once it is opened, the soymilk must be refrigerated. It will stay fresh for about 5 days. Soymilk is also sold as a powder, which must be mixed with water. Soymilk powder should be stored in the refrigerator or freezer. You can buy the powder and make your own so that you are sure there is no sweetener added.
Eden Foods -http://www.edenfoods.com/
WestSoy – http://www.westsoy.biz
Make unsweetened, plain varieties. Beware of "plain" varieties that still contain rice syrup, cane juice, and other sweeteners.

Soy Nuts - Halved, dry roasted (light) or whole, roasted in fat (dark). These also come flavored (Salsa, BBQ, Cheese, Onion, etc) and either salted or not. These are becoming extremely common and appear in grocery stores and drug stores now.

Soy Nut Butter - comes in low carb, unsweetened crunchy or low carb, unsweetened creamy varieties. Read labels carefully.
I.M. Healthy Soy Nut Butter - http://www.soynutbutter.com/product.html
SoSoya+ - http://www.portello.com

SoSoya+ - Dried soy product that comes in stir-fry sized "slices," at Trader Joe's. It's expensive, but it makes a fabulous stay-crunchy cereal. Vegetarian But Not Vegan: Tofu Pudding - from Plum Flower available in Asian grocery stores. It is apparently just like custard in consistency without any taste at all. You can add fruit or other tastes. It has gelatin so it isn't vegan.
SoSoya+ - http://www.portello.com

Thit Chay - pure soybeans - no other ingredient. It looks like pork rinds or cheese doodles and comes dark or light in 4 oz. bags that look like single serving potato chip bags. They are meant to be soaked in water and then used as a meat substitute in recipes.

Tempeh - soy tempeh rather than vegetable, rice, or other grain tempeh - may be eaten fresh out of the pack, or cooked in many ways, such as crumbled or stir fried in slices. Really good microwaved until crunchy.

Tofu - firm, medium, soft; fresh or cooked; blended into "yogurt", dip, or spread; fried, marinated, flavored, etc.

  Baked Tofu sold at Whole Foods, etc. Several flavors such as BBQ, Thai,etc.
  Fried Tofu is available in thick squares or triangles or thin strips and there are many brands.
  Tofu "Egg Salads" and other great imitation salads sold at various places. Check oil ingredients.

EXTRACTS - FLAVORINGS - SPICES - ALCOHOL-FREE, SUCROSE SUGAR-FREE

Bickford Flavors - http://www.bickfordflavors.com/
Or call 800-283-8322 and request a brochure.

Da Vinci's - http://www.davincigourmet.com/products
Splenda-Sweetened Flavored Syrups

Dolce - http://www.coffeeam.com/
Nutra-Sweetened Flavored Syrups

Frontier Coop - http://www.frontiercoop.com/
listed as "Natural Flavors"; or call 800-786-1388 and request a catalog.
Culinary spices, seasoning blends.

Nature's Flavors - http://www.naturesflavors.com/
bulk herbs and spices; Splenda-Sweetened Flavored Syrups -listed as "Flavor
Concentrates". Penzeys Spices - spices, herbs, and seasonings; gift boxes, specialty
spices; mills and containers

Spices Etc. - http://www.spicesetc.com/
herbs, spices, and seasonings; storage and usage tips; grinders,racks, gifts; Torani -
Splenda-Sweetened Flavored Syrups

BIBLIOGRAPHY

Alcoholics Anonymous, "*A.A. Conference Approved Statement on Drug Use,*" 1995, http://www.aa.org.

Alcoholics Anonymous, *Twelve Steps & Twelve Traditions*, 1953, http://www.aa.org.

Alcoholics Anonymous, Fourth Edition, 2001, http://www.aa.org. 2001.

Biology: Life on Earth with Physiology, 9th Ed., Teresa & Gerald Audesirk, Bruce E. Byers, Prentice-Hall, 2010.

Columbia Daily Tribune, "Sweet on Stevia: Sugar Substitute Gains Fans," March 23, 2008, http://archive.columbiatribune.com/2008/mar/20080323puls010.asp.

CEA-HOW (Compulsive Overeaters – HOW), CEA-HOW Food Plan, http://www.ceahow.org.

Cups & Scales Online Forum, cupsandscales-subscribe@yahoogroups.com, http://www.yahoogroups.com

Cups & Scales: Weighing & Measuring Food & Emotions, 2010, Partnerships for Community, N.Y., 2010.

Daniel J.W., Renwick A.G., Roberts A., Sims J. (2000). "The metabolic fate of sucralose in rats". Food Chem Tox 38 (S2): S115–S121, Science Direct, http://www.sciencedirect.com/science?_ob=ArticleURL&_udi=B6T6P-40NFPDF-F&_user=10&_coverDate=07%2F31%2F2000&_rdoc=1&_fmt=high&_orig=search&_s ort=d&_docanchor=&view=c&_acct=C000050221&_version=1&_urlVersion=0&_userid=10&md5=582f38e1216d11371f83c819302607b4.

DeNoon, Daniel J. Reviewed by Charlotte Grayson Mathis MD. "Drink More Diet Soda, Gain More Weight? Overweight Risk Soars 41% With Each Daily Can of Diet Soft Drink", WebMD Medical News, 2005, http://www.webmd.com/diet/news/20050613/drink-more-diet-soda-gain-more-weight.

Fletcher, Anthony, "Sucralose breakthrough could smash Tate & Lyle Monopoly," http://www.foodnavigator-usa.com/Financial-Industry/Sucralose-breakthrough-could-smash-Tate-Lyle-monopoly, January 12, 2006 .

Food Addiction: The Body Knows: Online Discussion Group, thebodyknows-yahoogroups.com; http://www.kaysheppard.com

Food Addicts Anonymous, "Food Addicts Anonymous Food Plan," http://www.foodaddictsanonymous.org, http://www.foodaddictsanonymous.org/faa-food-plan.

Food & Drug Administration, "No Calories... Sweet!," 2006 http://www.fda.gov/fdac/features/2006/406_sweeteners.html.

Food & Drug Administration, "FDA Website Guidance Doc
http://www.cfsan.fda.gov/~dms/grasguid.html#Q1

Greysheeters Anonymous Inc., http://www.greysheet.org

James, William, "The Varieties of Religious Experience," A Study in Human Nature
Being the Gifford Lectures on Natural Religion Delivered at Edinburgh in 1901-1902;
Public domain work, available at:
http://www2.hn.psu.edu/faculty/jmanis/wjames/Varieties-Rel-Exp.pdf
http://etext.virginia.edu/toc/modeng/public/JamVari.html

Mintz, Sidney, *Sweetness and Power,* 1985.

National Toxicology Program, Department of Health & Human Services, "Aspartame:
Questions & Answers; Study reaffirms safety of aspartame," 2002,
http://ntp-server.niehs.nih.gov/index.cfm?objectid=03614CBD-C0A2-C207-
C140B407A4043600;
http://ntp.niehs.nih.gov/ntp/Main_Pages/Transgen/AspartameTgProtocol.pdf.

Olney, JW, Farber, NB, Spitznagel E, Robins LN (November 1996). "Increasing brain
tumor rates: is there a link to aspartame?". J Neuropathol Exp Neurol. 55 (11): 1115–
23. doi:10.1097/00005072-199611000-00002. PMID 8939194

Overeaters Anonymous Inc."The Dignity of Choice" 2002, http://www.oa.org.

Recovery from Food Addiction, 2006,
recoveryfromfoodaddiction-subscribe@yahoogroups.com.

RuddCenter/Yale for Obesity & Food Addictions, http://www.ruddcenteryale.org.

Soffritti M, Belpoggi F, Degli Esposti D, Lambertini L, Tibaldi E, Rigano A (March
2006). "First experimental demonstration of the multipotential carcinogenic effects of
aspartame administered in the feed to Sprague-Dawley rats". Environ Health Perspect.
114 (3): 379–85. PMID 16507461.& PMC 1392232.
http:// www.ehponline.org/mem-bers/2005/8711/8711.html .

Swithers S.E., Davidson T.L. (2008). "A role for sweet taste: calorie predictive relations
in energy regulation by rats". Behav Neurosci 122 (1): 161–73.
http://psycnet.apa.org/?fa=main.doiLanding&doi=10.1037/0735-7044.122.1.161.

The Body Knows Online Discussion Group,
thebodyknows-subscribe@yahoogroups.com

Wanjek, Christopher, "Bitter Battle over Truth in Sweeteners," Live Science, May 2007,
http://www.livescience.com/health/070515_bad_sugar.html

Wikipedia, http://www.wikipedia.com.

Index

Recipes Index

DAIRY/PROTEIN
WITH DAIRY-FREE SUBSTITUTES

PROTEINS - ANIMAL & SOY

STARCH/GRAINS
INCLUDING BEANS/LEGUMES

STARCHY VEGETABLES

COOKED VEGETABLES

COOKED VEGETABLES
WITH PROTEIN

COOKED VEGETABLES
WITH PROTEIN
WITH STARCH/GRAIN

RAW VEGETABLES